RC860 L81

Columbia University
in the City of New York

College of Physicians and Surgeons

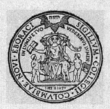

Reference Library

DISEASES OF THE COLON
AND THEIR SURGICAL TREATMENT

DISEASES OF THE COLON

AND THEIR SURGICAL TREATMENT

(FOUNDED ON THE JACKSONIAN ESSAY FOR 1909.)

BY

P. LOCKHART MUMMERY, F.R.C.S. Eng.,

B.A., M.B., B.C. CANTAB.,

*Jacksonian Prizeman and late Hunterian Professor, Royal College of Surgeons;
Senior Assistant Surgeon St. Mark's Hospital for Cancer, Fistula, and other Diseases
of the Rectum; and Senior Surgeon to Out-Patients, The Queen's Hospital
for Children, London*

ILLUSTRATED BY COLOURED AND OTHER PLATES,
AND NUMEROUS FIGURES IN THE TEXT, MANY OF WHICH ARE REPRODUCED
FROM THE AUTHOR'S SKETCHES

NEW YORK:
WILLIAM WOOD AND COMPANY.
MDCCCCX.

JOHN WRIGHT AND SONS LTD.
PRINTERS AND PUBLISHERS, BRISTOL.

PREFACE

UNTIL comparatively recently, diseases of the colon had received but scant attention, and with the exception of cancer and amœbic dysentery, little was known about the pathological conditions which occur in this portion of the alimentary tract. Everybody was treating constipation, but few knew anything about its causes. Within the last few years, however, chiefly as the result of better methods of diagnosis, our knowledge with regard to diseases of the colon has been much increased.

The subject is one of considerable importance, for everything points to the conclusion that diseases and abnormalities of the colon are becoming more frequent. This is probably to be attributed mainly to modern methods of dietary more than to any other factor. Among uncivilized races of mankind, the alimentary system has to digest and deal with food in which digestible and indigestible materials are about equally mixed. But under our present high state of civilization, foods, both animal and vegetable, are specially grown. The animals which supply our meat are specially bred and cared for to render it free from gristle, and the vegetables are cultivated to contain but little cellulose, and are further prepared, especially in the case of bread, to reduce this ingredient to the very minimum. Under these conditions, to which must often be added a sedentary occupation, the normal stimuli to peristalsis and digestion are to a large extent absent. And this, combined with other factors, one of which is the modern craze for patent aperient medicines, favours the production of disease in the colon.

This book is founded upon the Essay which was awarded the Jacksonian Prize for 1909 by the Royal College of Surgeons. In order to make it a practical and useful textbook, it has been necessary to make several additions to the original essay, and to condense some of the chapters dealing with rare conditions of the bowel. The earlier chapters are devoted to the anatomy and physiology of the colon, both in health and disease. The subject of diagnosis has been very thoroughly discussed, this being the factor presenting the greatest difficulty in dealing with disease when it attacks the colon. Special attention also has been paid to the effect of adhesions, and to chronic constipation and obstruction in their various forms. The different varieties of colitis are fully considered, as also are pericolitis and cancer.

The closing chapters of the book are devoted to a description of the various operations which may be performed on the colon.

I have to offer my best thanks to those friends who have kindly lent me blocks or illustrations.

P. L. M.

10, CAVENDISH PLACE, W.,
    May, 1910.

CONTENTS

CHAP.		PAGE
I.	THE ANATOMY AND DEVELOPMENT OF THE COLON	1
II.	PHYSIOLOGY OF THE COLON	13
III.	MORBID PHYSIOLOGY OF THE COLON	28
IV.	BACTERIOLOGY OF THE COLON	37
V.	METHODS OF DIAGNOSIS	41
VI.	CONGENITAL ABNORMALITIES OF THE COLON	58
VII.	VOLVULUS OF THE COLON	76
VIII.	ADHESIONS AND KINKING OF THE COLON	93
IX.	ENTEROPTOSIS OF THE TRANSVERSE COLON AND HERNIA OF THE COLON	107
X.	INTUSSUSCEPTION	114
XI.	CHRONIC MUCOUS OR MEMBRANOUS COLITIS	127
XII.	ULCERATIVE COLITIS	154
XIII.	PERICOLITIS	179
XIV.	TUBERCULOSIS OF THE COLON	201
XV.	CHRONIC CONSTIPATION AND FÆCAL IMPACTION	218
XVI.	SIMPLE STRICTURE OF THE COLON AND EMBOLISM OF THE MESOCOLIC VESSELS	233
XVII.	SIMPLE TUMOURS OF THE COLON	237
XVIII.	MALIGNANT DISEASE OF THE COLON	249
XIX.	TRAUMATISM	276
XX.	COLOTOMY	280
XXI.	APPENDICOSTOMY AND VALVULAR CÆCOSTOMY	294
XXII.	RESECTION AND ANASTOMOSIS OF THE COLON	302

DISEASES OF THE COLON.

Chapter I.

THE ANATOMY AND DEVELOPMENT OF THE COLON

THE ANATOMY OF THE COLON.

IN man, the colon starts in the right lower part of the abdomen, and passes up towards the liver, then across towards the spleen, and then downwards to reach the rectum. In most carnivorous animals, however, the cæcum lies under the liver, and the colon passes across and then down, having the shape of the letter L inverted, the colon thus being much shorter relatively than in man. In man the commencement of the colon forms a dilated pouch, called the cæcum, into which the small bowel opens by a valve-like opening. The caput coli may be looked upon almost as a second stomach, and Prof. Keith has pointed out that it corresponds both embryologically and anatomically to the stomach as regards function. It has the same relationship to the large bowel that the stomach has to the small bowel.

In some animals the cæcum or caput coli is the main organ of digestion; while in others, as in man, the stomach has this function.

In the iguana, the orang-utang, and some monkeys, the caput coli forms a separate viscus, with a valve between it and the ileum, and also between it and the colon (*Fig.* 1).

In the tapir, although there is no such perfect valve as exists in the iguana, there is a circular fold forming a definite division between the caput coli and the remainder of the colon.

In fishes there is no distinction into small and large bowel. In some animals, instead of the caput coli being dilated to form a cæcum, there are pouches connected with the large bowel which

THE ANATOMY

doubtless act similarly. Thus in the hyrax there are three so-called cæca, two paired and one single.

In the lemur (*Perodicticus patto*) a very curious arrangement exists. The colon is folded back upon itself twice, the folds being connected by a delicate mesentery.

In most animals the descending colon joins the rectum as a more or less straight tube, and there is no coil like the sigmoid flexure in man.

The colon extends from the ileocæcal valve to the rectosigmoidal junction. The exact position of this latter point has been rather uncertain, different writers having taken different points for the junction between the pelvic colon and the rectum; the correct anatomical point, however, is at the

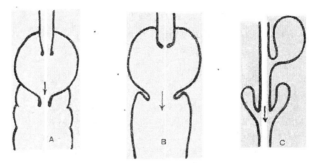

Fig. 1.—Diagrammatic representation of the Cæca of A, Iguana and Orang-utang; B, Tapir; and C, Hyrax.

position of what has by some observers been called the sigmoidorectal sphincter. There is at this point a distinct fold, or narrowing of the bowel lumen, which can easily be seen if the bowel is examined with the sigmoidoscope. This point corresponds roughly to the point at which the bowel becomes fixed.

The length of the colon varies considerably in different subjects. The average length is about 22 inches. Mr. Lockwood, from a study of dissecting-room subjects, found the usual length to be 22 inches, the longest he met with being 28 inches. Amussat found that it varied from 18 inches to 2 feet. The average length of the ascending colon is 8 inches, and that of the descending colon 8½ inches.

OF THE COLON

The most important parts of the colon from a surgical and pathological standpoint are the ileocæcal angle, the transverse colon, and the sigmoid flexure.

The cæcum and ascending colon are, as a rule, only partly covered by peritoneum, but exceptionally possess a mesentery ; the remainder of the colon has a more or less complete mesentery.

The Ileocæcal Valve.—This varies considerably in different animals, though in all its object is the same, namely, to prevent regurgitation of the contents of the cæcum into the ileum.

In many animals an oblique opening is depended on, somewhat similar to the opening of the ureter into the bladder in man (*Fig.* 2).

In others, notably in the iguana, tapir, and many monkeys, the valve is at the extremity of a conical papilla-like projection

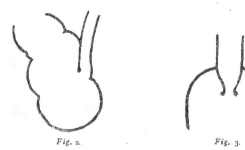

Fig. 2.   Fig. 3.

of the ileum into the cæcum, any tendency towards regurgitation resulting in the sides of the ileocæcal opening being pushed together (*Fig.* 3).

In man, however, and in some animals, there is a definite muscular sphincter, and it is upon this, rather than upon the formation of the opening, that its integrity as a valve depends. In the bear, ferret, and hedgehog there is no sphincter, and the mechanical advantages of an oblique opening are depended upon.

The ileocæcal sphincter in man is much better developed than in any of the lower animals. Elliott proved that there is a true sphincter in the cat, and was able to investigate its action. He found that stimulation of the sympathetic nerves causes contraction of the sphincter, though at the same time inhibiting the circular fibres in the ileum and colon adjoining. In the cat these constrictor fibres come from the 13th dorsal and 1st and 2nd lumbar roots.

Both anæmia and the application of adrenalin caused the same effect as stimulation of the sympathetic, i.e., constriction.

Removal of the cord abolished the power to keep apart the contents of the ileum and colon.

Blood-vessels of the Colon.—The arteries of the colon run in a circular direction round the bowel from the mesenteric border to the free margin, the vessels lying roughly parallel to one another. The arteries of the wall of the colon do not anastomose freely with one another, and in consequence, if care is not taken when resecting portions of the large bowel, the blood-supply is easily damaged, and sloughing results. For this reason it is

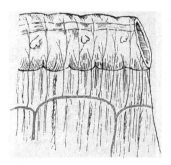

Fig. 4.—Diagram to show the way in which the arteries pass from the arterial arcades to the colon wall.

a good plan, when dividing the bowel, to make the division slightly oblique, so that rather more is cut away at the free margin than on the attached border (*Fig.* 4). This insures the whole of the edge of the divided bowel having a good blood-supply. The different parts of the colon differ somewhat as regards the arrangement of the blood-vessels. In the greater part of the colon the arteries anastomose by a series of loops just before reaching the bowel; these loops lie close to the mesenteric border of the bowel and form a free anastomosis. In the sigmoid flexure, however, the arteries usually anastomose nearer the base of the mesocolon, and then pass straight to the bowel; so that there is, as a rule, no free anastomosis to preserve the blood-supply of the colon when the mesosigmoid is cut close to its bowel attachment. This is an important point to be considered when planning a resection of any part of the pelvic colon.

There are three branches of the superior mesenteric artery to the colon—the ileocolic, the colica dextra, and the colica media. The cæcum is supplied by branches from all these three arteries.

Mr. Jamieson and Mr. Dobson* found that the colica dextra

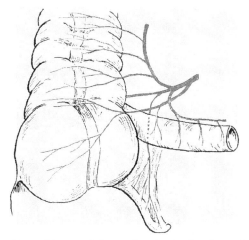

Fig. 5.—Diagram of the cæcal angle, showing ileocæcal artery and its branches.

artery is a direct branch of the superior mesenteric artery in less than 50 per cent of cases. In about 30 per cent it is a branch of the ileocolic.

The colica media artery arises from the superior mesenteric, just below the lower border of the pancreas, and passes downwards across the superior mesenteric vein to enter the transverse mesocolon. Half-way to the colon it divides into two branches; these again divide near the colon, forming a series of arcades from which branches pass to the colon wall. The largest of these arcades lies one or two fingers' breadth from the bowel along the left two-thirds of the transverse colon, and encloses

---

* *Trans. Roy. Soc. Med.*, Feb. 9, 1909.

THE ANATOMY

a large area of mesocolon containing very few vessels. The end of this arcade anastomoses freely with a branch of the inferior mesenteric artery.

The inferior mesenteric artery leaves the aorta behind the duodenum and passes downwards across the aorta and left psoas muscle. It gives off the colica sinistra and sigmoidea arteries to the colon. The colica sinistra, which is the most important, leaves the parent trunk close to the latter's origin

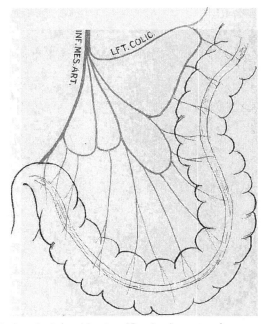

Fig. 6.—Blood supply of the pelvic colon. Note that the anastomosis occurs some way from the bowel wall, and is destroyed by cutting the mesocolon close to the bowel.

from the aorta. It passes upwards across the kidney towards the splenic flexure, where it divides to anastomose on the one hand with the colica media artery and supply the left part of the transverse colon, and on the other with the sigmoidea arteries to supply the descending colon. There are usually three or four sigmoid arteries which anastomose with each other by short arcades; the lowest anastomoses with the superior hæmorrhoidal artery.

OF THE COLON

The method of this last anastomosis is important, as pointed out by Jamieson and Dobson (*Fig.* 7).

Lymphatics of the Colon.—The lymphatics follow roughly the arteries and veins. Jamieson and Dobson, who have made a careful study of the lymphatic arrangements of the colon, divide the lymphatic glands into the following groups :

The epicolic glands, which lie on the intestinal wall and in the appendices epiploicæ. These are particularly numerous in the pelvic colon. They drain into the next two groups.

The paracolic glands, which lie along the inner edge of the gut in the mesenteric attachment ; and

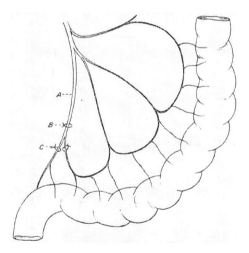

Fig. 7.—A, Inferior mesenteric artery ; B, ligature without destroying anastomosis ; C, ligatures breaking the anastomosis. [JAMIESON and DOBSON, *Proc. Roy. Soc. Med.*, Vol. 2, 1909.]

The intermediate groups, which lie along the arteries and at their junctions.

In addition to these groups there are the *main groups* into which all the foregoing drain. There are three main groups or chains which can be distinguished, though any such classification is in a sense arbitrary. Nine isolated groups of glands are common.

There is the middle colic group, which lies on the middle colic artery at the foot of the transverse mesocolon.

The left colic group lies partly on the horizontal portion of

THE ANATOMY

the artery near its origin, and partly on the terminal portion of the mesenteric vein. These glands drain into the superior mesenteric, cœliac, and lumbar glands. The inferior mesenteric group lies on the stem of the inferior mesenteric artery; its glands drain into, and may almost be considered as forming part of, the lumbar glands. It is this chain of glands which drains

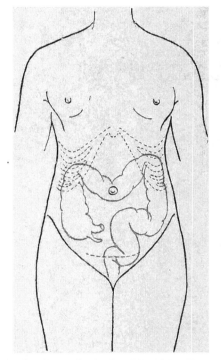

Fig. 8.—Diagram showing the relation of the colon to the abdominal parietes.

the pelvic colon. It is important to notice that some of the lymphatics of the left half of the transverse colon drain into the glands at the hilum of the spleen, passing *via* the gastrocolic omentum.

Jamieson and Dobson found evidence of a communication between the lymphatic and venous systems in the abdomen, though they were unable to ascertain at what particular point this occurred.

PLATE I

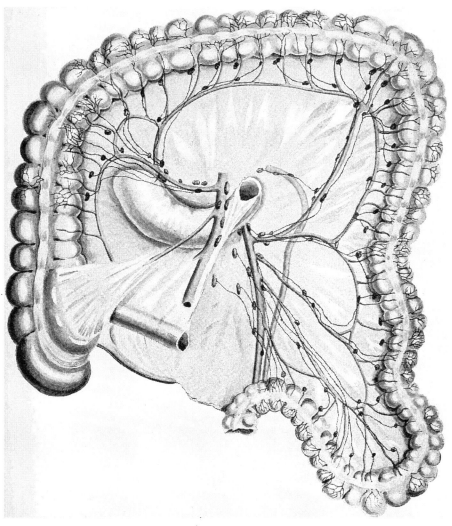

THE LYMPHATICS OF THE COLON

(JAMIESON and DOBSON, *Proc. Roy. Soc. Med.* Vol. ii., 1909.)

OF THE COLON

The Sigmoid Flexure or Pelvic Colon.—This is the mobile portion of the colon, which is situated between the straight and fixed descending colon and the fixed rectum, and the average length is 17½ inches. It forms a loop which, in a normal man in the erect position, lies forward and falls across the front of the rectum, lying partly behind the bladder or uterus, and partly in the left iliac fossa. It has a long mesentery, which is fan-shaped, having a short attachment 3 inches long, situated along a line from the left sacro-iliac synchondrosis to the mid-line of the sacrum.

There is normally a slight kink or angle where the pelvic colon joins the rectum, but this is prevented by the mesentery from becoming an obstruction. When the mesosigmoid is abnormal or has become stretched, this kink is much exaggerated and may cause a considerable degree of obstruction.

THE DEVELOPMENT OF THE COLON.

The colon begins to be differentiated from the rest of the alimentary canal about the sixth week of intra-uterine life.

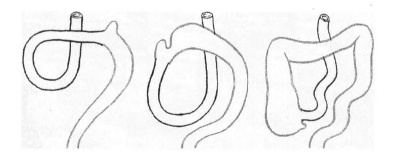

Fig 9.—Diagram of three stages in the development of the colon, showing how the cæcum passes from the left to the right side of the abdomen, and then downwards into the right iliac fossa. The cæcum and colon are coloured, and the small bowel black.

The cæcum first appears as a lateral protrusion of the alimentary tube. This protrusion forms just beyond the vitelline duct, and gradually increases in size except at its blind extremity, which remains narrow and becomes the vermiform appendix. As the alimentary canal increases in length it forms a loop, the lower limb of which forms the colon, which thus comes to be placed transversely in the peritoneal cavity lying in front of the commencement of the small intestine.

In the third and fourth month of intra-uterine life the cæcum lies at about the centre of the abdomen, while the remainder of the colon lies as a curved tube in the left hypochondriac and left iliac regions, attached by a mesentery to the front of the spine.

As the alimentary canal increases in length and the loop enlarges, the cæcum and upper part of the colon are carried upwards and to the left, and then over to the right, so that the cæcum comes to lie under the liver in the right hypochondriac region. At this stage the colon resembles that found in the dog, cat, and other carnivorous mammalia in whom there is no ascending colon.

Later still, the cæcum passes downward towards the right iliac fossa. In the eighth-month fœtus the cæcum is just below the right iliac crest, and the colon forms the typical inverted U of man. The causes of the descent of the cæcum into the right iliac fossa are somewhat uncertain, but it has been pointed out by Mr. Lockwood that in the eighth-month fœtus there is a band of peritoneum passing from the right testis to the cæcum close to the termination of the ileum, and he has suggested it as probable that the cæcum is carried down into the right iliac fossa by the descent of the testicle. Lockwood found that in the female fœtus there is a similar relationship between the right ovary and the cæcum.

The probability of this view is much increased by the fact that imperfect descent of the cæcum is frequently accompanied by undescended testicle.

Under abnormal conditions the colon may be arrested at any stage of its development, in which case the fœtal condition will persist after birth. When this occurs it is generally the result of adhesions having formed to fix the colon and prevent its descent. Evidence of these adhesions, generally formed as the result of some inflammatory condition during intra-uterine life, are usually to be found if carefully looked for.

It will be obvious that if the progress of the colon is arrested, it may be found in any of the following positions, according to the period at which arrest took place.

If arrested very early, the cæcum may be outside the abdomen, and the colon pass as an almost straight tube to the rectum. The cæcum may lie in the central or left upper portion of the abdominal cavity, and the transverse and ascending portions of the colon be missing.

The cæcum may lie under the liver in the right hypochondriac region, so that the condition found is that normally present in the dog, there being no ascending colon.

Or the cæcum may have partly descended, but not reached the right iliac fossa, the ascending colon being very short.

Cases are recorded in which all these conditions have persisted as the result of arrested development, and will be referred to in dealing with congenital abnormalities of the colon.

The Development of the Mesentery.—At first, the whole alimentary tract possesses a mesentery, which increases in length with the growth of the intestine, except in the case

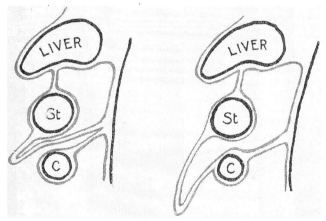

Fig. 10.—Diagrams showing the development of the great omentum. The peritoneum is shown in red. (St.) Stomach. (C) Colon.

of the duodenum and the ascending and descending colon. The cæcum and the ascending and descending colon, as they grow, push themselves between the layers of the mesentery so that the latter becomes to a large extent obliterated, and these portions of the colon normally lose their mesentery by the time development is complete.

While the colon is passing across the abdomen to reach the right hypochondriac region, it possesses a common mesentery with the small intestine, and if it is arrested in this stage of

12 THE DEVELOPMENT OF THE COLON

development it retains this arrangement of the mesentery. In cases of undescended cæcum there is generally a long mesentery to the right-hand portion of the colon, which enables it to become twisted and form a volvulus.

The mesentery of the transverse colon is at first entirely separate from the great omentum or mesogastrium (the original mesentery of the stomach) lying transversely behind it, but the two membranes fuse about the fourth month, so that the transverse colon comes to lie in the posterior surface of the great omentum (*Fig.* 10).

Chapter II.

PHYSIOLOGY OF THE COLON.

FUNCTIONS OF THE LARGE INTESTINE.

Re-absorption of Water.—One of the most important functions of the colon is to prevent loss of water from the body. By means of the re-absorption of water from the intestinal contents which occurs in the colon, the body is protected against the loss of fluid which would otherwise take place, and which, under conditions different from those usually existing at the present day, would seriously prejudice the chances of the individual in the struggle for existence. Digestion and absorption cannot be carried out in the absence of water, and most animals, including man, must under uncivilized conditions be very dependent upon the retention of moisture or fluid within the tissues for long periods without the necessity of replenishment. To this end it is an obvious economy to remove the moisture from the excreta before their dejection from the body. It seems reasonable to suppose that, in the process of evolution, material advantage would accrue to those animals which were best able to preserve their fluids ; and it is quite obvious that a considerable loss of water would occur if the dejecta were as fluid as the contents of the ileum. In birds the body fluids are even better preserved than in mammals, for the uric acid is got rid of in a semi-solid state with the dejecta of the bowel.

This is a distinct economy of the amount of fluid, and would seem to be of advantage in lessening the weight which has to be supported in the air, while, at the same time, doing away with the necessity for frequent replenishment.

In cases where, for the relief of some diseased condition, a right inguinal colotomy has been performed so that the dejecta escape at the termination of the ileum instead of first passing through the colon, the patient always suffers considerably from thirst, and it is quite obvious that a great waste of body fluid is occurring.

Absorption of Food Constituents.—In addition to its function of removing moisture from the excreta, there can be no doubt that the colon absorbs some of the food constituents of its contents. There is abundant evidence that the walls of the cæcum and colon can absorb fats, and it seems almost certain that carbohydrates and even proteids can also be absorbed.

There has recently been much dispute as to the value of the colon, and there are not wanting those who maintain that we should be better and healthier if we possessed no colon. The fact that human beings can live without a colon is, however, no proof of its uselessness, and at present the evidence brought forward to prove that the colon is a useless and effete portion of the alimentary tract is anything but convincing. Under conditions of modern civilization it is undoubtedly possible for human beings to live without a colon, and perhaps even for it not to be missed; but man was not designed to live in a London flat with servants and a banking account, and this can hardly, therefore, be taken as an argument that the colon is useless.

NERVE SUPPLY OF THE COLON.

The nerves governing the movements of the colon are derived from the spinal cord and the plexuses of the sympathetic. The nerve fibres from the cord pass through the sympathetic plexuses and ganglia, and not direct from the cord, with the exception of the rectum and lower part of the sigmoid flexure, which receive their fibres from the first three sacral nerves via the hypogastric plexus.

There are also fibres from the splanchnics and from the vagi which reach the colon, as there is distinct evidence of the movements of the colon being affected by central nerve impulses. Thus, diarrhœa and a desire to defæcate is undoubtedly produced in some individuals by emotions such as fear or nervousness, while the movements of the colon which produce borborygmi have always been supposed to result from emotion, the expression "the bowels of compassion" having its origin in this belief.

The movements of the bowel normally result from reflex nerve impulses, originating probably in Auerbach's plexus lying between the two muscular coats of the colon, and the initial impulse originates from causes within the bowel, usually either chemical or tactile. Heat, however, may cause peristalsis, though no sensation of warmth is produced.

I have noted that the introduction of warm water into the colon in cases of appendicostomy produces immediate and sometimes violent peristalsis much more readily than the introduction of cold water. The same fact is also seen where a draught of hot liquid is used to promote the action of the bowels.

Sensory Nerves of the Colon.—The normal mucous membrane of the colon does not possess ordinary tactile sensation.

Damage or injury to the colon does not cause pain directly, though it may do so by the secondary consequences produced, such as peritonitis or peristalsis.

I have studied the effect of injury to the colon in animals, and although no attempt was made to produce pain, as the animals were under full anæsthesia, it was possible, by observing the effect upon the blood-pressure, to notice whether any effect upon the central nervous system was produced through afferent impulses reaching the higher centres from the injured area. The blood-pressure readily responds to any injury to sensory nerve-endings, and therefore this method gives probably just as reliable results as would be the case were an attempt made to produce pain, and as I shall be able to show, the results obtained correspond with observations which have been made in man.

I found that an injury such as crushing or ligaturing the wall of the colon produced no effect at all, providing the mesentery was not touched. This was the same both for the visceral peritoneum and the mucous membrane. A similar injury to the parietal peritoneum or to the mesentery of the colon did produce an effect upon the blood-pressure.

In a man who has had a colotomy performed it is possible to confirm this. The usual practice is to open the bowel some two days after the operation, and when this is done it is noticeable that cutting the bowel wall does not cause pain or any other sensation. When abdominal operations are performed under local anæsthesia, it is found necessary to anæsthetize the parietal peritoneum as well as the skin. Directly the parietal peritoneum is touched, if it has not been previously anæsthetized, the patient complains of pain; but the colon can be manipulated or operated upon without causing pain and without being anæsthetized, providing the mesocolon is not damaged or dragged upon; either of the latter will cause pain or uncomfortable sensations.

The pain produced by peritonitis or distention must be attributed to the parietal peritoneum and mesocolon.

NERVE SUPPLY

Violent peristalsis undoubtedly produces severe pain, and this must probably be attributed to the bowel wall itself, and is due to violent muscular contraction.

The mucous membrane of the rectum for about an inch above the muco-cutaneous junction is markedly sensitive to tactile or painful stimuli. Any injury to the mucous membrane in this area can be felt and, if severe enough, will cause pain. Ulcers in this situation are also painful, while higher up they do not cause pain directly. Injury to the mucous membrane in the higher part of the rectum and in the colon does not cause pain.

From the consideration of these facts I was led to study the

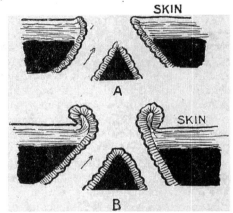

Fig. 11.—Diagrammatic section of a colotomy opening. The control obtained will be better in A than in B, owing to the greater amount of sensation at the edge. The mucous membrane is shown shaded.

condition of sensation at the opening of an artificial anus. As has already been mentioned, no sensation is present in the mucous membrane of a recent artificial anus; but I found that after a certain time the mucous membrane at the edge of the opening becomes sensitive, so that in an old artificial anus, any injury to the mucous membrane near its junction with the skin produces pain, and tactile sensation is present.

The time necessary for this change to take place varies considerably. It does not usually occur under six months, and often not till much later; while in some cases it does not appear to occur at all.

The following are instances in which I have observed this development of sensation in the mucous membrane at the orifice of an artificial anus.

In the case of a woman of 48, who had had her rectum and half the sigmoid flexure removed for cancer by abdomino-perineal excision, the centre of the sigmoid flexure having been brought down and stitched to the skin at the anal margin, I found, a year later, that she could feel the presence of fæces in the new rectum, and they caused a desire to evacuate. If the mucous membrane within the anal canal was nipped with forceps, she complained of pain.

A man, aged 34, who had had a similar operation performed, complained of pain if the mucous membrane was nipped, and could feel the presence of fæces in the rectum a year and a half after the operation.

In the case of a woman, aged 33, who had had a complete excision of the rectum performed for cancer, and the sigmoid flexure brought down and stitched to the skin, I found that she had well-marked sensation a year later in the mucous membrane of the new rectum.

In a case of colotomy, a year and a half after operation—man, aged 60—the patient could feel the presence of fæces in the colon above the opening, and complained of pain if the mucous membrane near the orifice was pinched.

In a man of 33 with a colotomy, the same condition was noticed nine months after operation.

PERISTALSIS.

The Effect of its Contents upon Peristalsis of the Colon.—The normal stimulus which produces peristalsis in the colon arises from the presence of something within the bowel. Peristalsis does not normally occur in an empty colon, and the normal stimulus is the presence of a certain quantity of fæcal material within it.

There is good reason to suppose that the contraction of the unstriped muscle fibre of the intestine takes place normally only as the result of local stimulus. Rapidly increasing tension, usually distention, is another normal stimulus to contraction.

Experimentally, peristalsis of the colon may be produced artificially in several ways. The introduction of irritant fluids into the colon will induce peristalsis, but in my experiments their effect was not well marked. Such substances as alcohol, solution of nicotine, acids, etc., were introduced through a small cannula, and the effect upon the colon was then carefully watched. Occasionally slow waves of peristalsis occurred and continued for a short time, but more often no effect resulted. In these experiments the animals were under full anæsthesia, which tended to prevent peristalsis; but this fallacy could be got over to some extent by the previous injection of a suitable dose of ergot or ernutin, which makes the colon more sensitive to anything which will cause peristalsis.

Large doses of ergot injected subcutaneously cause considerable and prolonged contraction of the muscular wall of the colon, and this may be used as a means of combating paralysis of the colon in cases of peritonitis or meteorism, and will be referred to in discussing the treatment of these conditions.

Experimentally, by far the readiest means of producing peristalsis in the colon is by stretching the bowel wall, i.e., by distention. In my experiments this was done by distending a portion of the organ either with air or with warm water. The air or water was pumped into the colon with a 10-cc. glass syringe, through a hypodermic needle pushed slantwise through the bowel wall.

Distention with water was found to act rather better than air. As soon as the bowel was distended, strong peristaltic waves commenced in the distended area, and continued until the distention was got rid of. It was found that distention in this way produced peristalsis more readily than any other form of stimulus.

A local injury to the mucosa, or bowel wall, such as a nip with the end of a pair of forceps, always resulted in a peristaltic contraction, of the circular fibres chiefly. The contraction occurred slowly, did not commence immediately, and took from thirty seconds to a minute before it was complete, when a narrow ring of contraction had occurred narrowing the lumen to about one-sixth of its normal diameter.

The contraction from such a traumatic stimulus was always local, and did not spread in either direction or cause waves of peristalsis. This very slow response to traumatic stimulus of the colon is different from what occurs in the small bowel, where the resultant contraction is the same, but occurs much more rapidly.

We have evidence that peristalsis of the colon can be induced by chemicals or other substances introduced into the bowel. Substances such as calomel, castor oil, etc., introduced into the colon through an appendicostomy opening, cause well-marked peristalsis ; but this action is not so marked as if given by the mouth.

Distention with water introduced through an appendicostomy opening rapidly produces peristalsis, the fluid being evacuated at the anus in about two minutes, thus showing that very active peristalsis must have occurred.

An interesting fact I have noticed is, that the introduction of a solution of bile—fel bovinum of the British Pharmacopœia—into the cæcum through an appendicostomy opening has a marked effect in stimulating peristalsis of the colon.

Among the abnormal causes of contraction are :—
1. The presence of a foreign body.
2. Inflammation or any local irritative lesion.
3. Certain drugs or foods, notably ergot.
4. Excess of carbonic acid in the blood ; this is well seen in the contraction occurring in the intestine in asphyxial conditions.

Simple complete obstruction of the bowel lumen does not cause peristalsis providing the bowel is empty. Accumulation of fæcal material above the obstruction, however, soon occurs, and as a result of this, rather than of the obstruction itself, violent peristalsis soon ensues.

If the obstruction is complete, the peristalsis after a time ceases, and is followed by paresis of the gut wall.

If the obstruction is incomplete or intermittent, hypertrophy and increased activity of the muscular wall ultimately develops.

The time after a meal at which food commences to pass from the small intestine through the ileocæcal valve into the cæcum is difficult to ascertain, and probably it varies considerably according to the individual and the nature of the food.

Sir William Macewen was able to observe the passage of food through the ileocæcal valve in a patient, the anterior wall of whose cæcum had been destroyed by an explosion. He found that in one or two hours after a meal, chyme in small quantities began to pass the ileocæcal valve.

Dr. Hertz, who made careful X-ray observations upon human beings who had previously been given large doses of bismuth, found that the first appearance of a shadow indicating the presence of food in the cæcum occurred in from $3\frac{1}{2}$ to 5 hours after a meal ; the average time of a number of observations being

$4\frac{3}{8}$ hours. This is considerably longer than Macewen found: but in Hertz's observations it is obvious that no shadow would appear till a fair quantity of chyme had passed into the cæcum.

No movements occur in the empty colon, but as soon as the cæcum has become slightly distended, slow peristaltic movements occur in the cæcum and colon up to about the centre of the transverse colon.

At first these movements are chiefly antiperistaltic, a series of waves of contraction, one following the other, occurring in an antiperistaltic direction from the centre of the transverse colon backwards towards the ileocæcal valve. The presence of antiperistalsis in the colon was first discovered accidentally by Jacobi. Several writers have denied that antiperistalsis occurs normally, but as I shall be able to show, it is quite certain that it does. Antiperistalsis was observed by Elliott and Barclay-Smith in cats and rats.

Cannon made observations with the X rays upon cats who had been given large doses of bismuth in their food, the cats having previously been given nothing for twelve hours, and the bowels emptied with castor oil. He confirmed Jacobi's observation. Antiperistaltic waves could be seen to start near the end of the transverse colon and pass backwards towards the cæcum. The first period of antiperistalsis lasted from two to eight minutes, there was then an interval of from fifteen to forty-five minutes, when the antiperistaltic waves again occurred.

The rate of contraction observed by Cannon was about eleven waves in two minutes.

Waves of segmentation and resegmentation were observed by him in one case in the ascending colon, the segmentation being followed by antiperistalsis.

No leakage past the ileocæcal valve in the reverse direction as the result of antiperistalsis was observed.

Dr. Hertz, in a series of similar experiments carried out upon healthy men, observed the same phenomena of antiperistalsis.

I have done several experiments upon cats with the object of observing the movements of the colon. The animals were kept anæsthetized with ether in a warm saline tank, and the colon exposed. It was found possible in this way to keep the bowel warm and active for an hour or more, while at the same time it could be carefully watched. To induce peristalsis warm

PERISTALSIS

water was injected into the colon with a hypodermic syringe until slight distention had been produced.

The antiperistaltic waves could be well seen. First, a ring of contraction occurred in the transverse colon and began to move

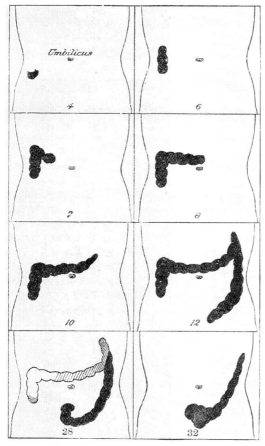

Fig. 12.—Series of colon skiagrams in a normal individual. The numbers represent the hours after a bismuth breakfast was taken. [*Constipation*, Dr. HERTZ: by kind permission *Oxf. Med. Pub.*]

along towards the cæcum. After it had gone about an inch, another occurred and followed it, and so on, so that a long series of rings of contraction could be observed passing towards the ileocæcal valve, where they disappeared. The antiperistaltic movement was in no case carried into the ileum. After these antiperistaltic waves have continued for some minutes, slow segmentation occurs in the colon. Broad bands of contraction occur at definite intervals along the colon, and remain for a minute or more, then they relax, and others take their place at intermediate positions.

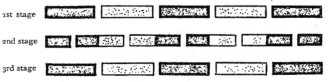

Fig. 13.—Diagram of segmentation. Notice that although the material is divided and re-divided, no movement takes place in either direction.

This segmentation may be followed by more antiperistalsis, but sooner or later slow peristaltic waves in the normal direction occur, tending to pass the contents on towards the descending colon. The object of the antiperistaltic waves is evidently to mix up the contents of the colon, and to bring them intimately into contact with the bowel wall. Whether this is simply to allow of as much moisture as possible being removed from the chyme, or whether it indicates digestive absorption, as occurring in the cæcum, it is not possible to say. It is certain that fat is absorbed in the colon, because olive oil introduced into the cæcum or rectum is absorbed in small quantities ; and in 1814, Sir Everard Home pointed out that, whereas fat could be extracted from the contents of the cæcum in ducks, it could not be found in the contents of the lower bowel.

Cannon observed that if enemas were administered to cats, antiperistalsis occurred, and the material reached the cæcum, while if the enema was a very large one, a considerable quantity was forced backwards through the ileocæcal valve into the ileum.

In no instance has antiperistalsis been observed in the ileum, and it probably does not normally occur.

The peristaltic waves in the descending colon and sigmoid are slow forward movements, and antiperistalsis is not observed here.

Dr. Hertz found that it took about $4\frac{1}{2}$ hours for food to pass from the cæcum to the splenic flexure, and about 16 to 17 hours to pass from there to the lower end of the sigmoid flexure. He found that it took 6 hours to pass along the sigmoid flexure. The sigmoid flexure is the normal reservoir for fæcal material before dejection, and not, as is often supposed, the rectum. The normal function of the rectum is only as an expulsive organ, and the presence of fæces within the rectum normally gives rise to an immediate desire to defæcate. In animals in a state of nature this desire is immediately followed by the act of defæcation, as is also often the case in paralyzed persons. The necessities of civilization, which prevents the possibility of defæcation taking place directly the desire occurs, has necessitated the use of the sigmoid, and sometimes of the rectum, as a reservoir for fæcal material in the intervals between defæcation. The rectum of a normal individual, however, does not contain fæces except just before and during the act of defæcation. I have examined the rectum of a great number of patients, and in the large majority of healthy individuals, that is to say those who are not habitually constipated, the rectum is empty. It is only as the result of habitual constipation and carelessness that the rectum becomes a reservoir for fæcal material.

Dr. Hertz, who carried out a number of observations with the X rays upon patients suffering from chronic constipation, found that the cause of the delay in the movements of the colon varied considerably in different cases. Thus, it might be that the fæcal current was slower in all parts of the colon, or only in one part. In some cases it was only in the sigmoid and rectum, while in others it was in the transverse colon, the passage through the sigmoid and rectum taking place in the normal time.

Reversal Experiments.—By this is meant resecting a portion of the large bowel, turning it round, and sewing it in the reverse position.

These experiments have been done by numerous observers, notably by Beers and Eggers, Balance, Edmunds, Kelling, and Hess, the object being to ascertain if antiperistalsis occurs in the colon. The best proofs of this now well-established fact are, however, the X-ray experiments on animals and human beings.

In those cases in which, after union had taken place, the abdomen of the animal was opened, and the peristalsis in the reversed loop watched, as in the experiments of Beers and Eggers, peristaltic waves could be seen to occur in the reversed loop in the same direction as in the normal colon, the peristaltic wave passing through the reversed loop to the bowel below it. This was observed on several occasions in different animals. It was almost constantly found that the bowel above the reversed loop was much dilated, often for a considerable distance, and contained foreign bodies, such as stones or fæcal concretions. There was also considerable hypertrophy of the bowel wall above the reversed loop.

These experiments show that the reversed loop causes an undoubted obstruction to the intestinal flux, but that the flow is re-established and becomes in time more or less normal.

The experiment of Murchison, in which nearly all the small gut was reversed, and yet the animal defæcated normally and lived three weeks, and similar experiments of Beers and Eggers on the small and large gut, go much further to prove antiperistalsis.

CONTENTS OF THE COLON.

Normally, the contents of the cæcum and ascending colon are liquid or semi-fluid, while those of the sigmoid flexure are solid.

Mucus.—Mucus is a normal content of the colon, and is freely secreted by its walls. Macewen observed the secretion of mucus by the walls of the cæcum, and found that it began just *before* the chyme passed from the ileum into the cæcum.

A considerable amount of mucus is normally present in the fæces, but not in sufficient quantities to be obvious. In certain diseased states, however, an abnormal amount of secretion occurs. This is notably the case in chronic mucous and membranous colitis, in which very large quantities of mucus are passed "per anum." In membranous colitis, the mucus may be in the form of complete casts of the bowel. The walls of these tubular casts, which may be a foot or more in length and conform to the shape of the colon, are laminated, and consist of mucus and epithelial casts.

Microscopically, they are structureless ; and, chemically, they consist of mucus.

Much importance has been attached to these casts, and their presence in the stools has been attributed to a disease called membranous colitis. The casts are simply the normal mucus of the colon secreted in abnormal quantities which, for some reason, has remained on the surface of the mucosa and become solidified there, so that a complete cast of the bowel in mucus has formed

THE COLON

which, sooner or later, has become separated and dejected in its entirety.

Excessive secretion of mucus will result from any irritative condition of the colon, such as chronic inflammation, cancer, polypus, intussusception, etc.

There does not seem to be any sound reason for attaching special significance to the form in which the mucus is present in the stools.

Fat in the Stools.—A certain amount of fat is normally present in the stools in most individuals. The amount which is absorbed during the passage of the food through the intestine is very limited, and any excess of fat in the diet will, in almost all cases, lead to an excess of fat in the stools.

If mineral fats are included in the diet, such as petroleum or vaseline, they are not absorbed at all, and re-appear again in the stools.

Most animal and mineral fats are liquid at body temperature, and, consequently, if there be an excess of fat in the stools, the latter will be semi-solid or liquid, and this fact may be made use of in the treatment of some varieties of constipation.

It also affords us a most valuable method of keeping the stools liquid and soft after an operation in which the colon has been resected, or an anastomosis has been performed, and we wish to avoid any possibility of strain due to solid faecal material being thrown upon a recent wound in the bowel wall.

Intestinal Sand.—Intestinal sand is occasionally present in the faeces as an abnormal constituent, and may cause bleeding and severe pain, owing to the traumatism of the mucosa involved in its passage along the intestinal tract. The origin of this sand has not been ascertained, but it closely corresponds to the uric acid gravel passed in urine. When first passed it is red in colour, but soon becomes black when kept in contact with the air. Its composition is as follows:—

Organic matter	30–70 per cent.
Inorganic matter	Calcium phosphate 98 per cent.
	Magnesium ⎫
	Iron ⎬ A trace
	Calcium oxalate ⎪
	Silica ⎭

I had one patient who passed as much as two ounces in twenty-four hours; but usually there is much less than this.

Other Abnormal Contents.—In cases of intestinal obstruction, the contents of the colon become altered. This is probably due to two causes :—

1. Abnormal retention of the contents allows excessive and abnormal fermentation to occur.
2. The normal absorption and secretion of the bowel-wall being arrested, abnormal substances are able to form.

Nesbitt, who produced intestinal obstruction artificially in dogs, found that highly poisonous substances were formed in the obstructed loops of bowel. The most notable of these were neurin and cholin, both of which are not present in the normal bowel contents.

These substances are of the nature of what are known as toxins, and it is the absorption of such toxins through the damaged bowel-wall and their entry into the blood-stream which is one of the principal causes of death in cases of intestinal obstruction.

Some experiments carried out by Clairmont and Ranzi prove the extremely poisonous nature of these toxins. They found that, while the filtrate from the contents of a normal intestine produced no harmful effects when injected into animals, a similar filtrate prepared from the contents of a loop of strangulated bowel produced serious, and often fatal, results when injected.

The normal fæces are solid or semi-solid, depending on the dietary, and to some extent the personal habits, of the individual.

Fluid fæces are always abnormal, and the result of some disturbance of the digestive functions, or of some pathological process.

Diarrhœa may be of two kinds : (*a*) Lienteric diarrhœa, in which the fluidity is due to insufficient absorption of the fluids ingested ; (*b*) Excessive secretion by the walls of the colon.

Lienteric Diarrhœa may result from increased activity of the muscular wall of the colon, so that the contents, which are fluid on reaching the cæcum, are hurried on before there has been time for the fluid constituents to be absorbed ; or it may be due to a loss of the normal absorptive power of the mucosa.

The commonest pathological cause of diarrhœa is certainly *Excessive Secretion* by the mucosa of the colon, due to irritative or inflammatory conditions. But insufficient absorption is also present in most cases.

The colour of the fæces is almost entirely dependent upon the constituents of the food, or to the presence of bile or blood in the stools.

The normal colour of the fæces is due to bile. Light-coloured or yellow stools may result from less bile than normal, or from excess of fats.

A normal stool is slightly acid. The acidity is often increased when there is inflammation or increased fermentation in the colon.

REFERENCES.

CANNON.—*Amer. Jour. of Phys.* Jan. 1904.
ELLIOTT and BARCLAY SMITH.—*Jour. of Phys.* 1904, p. 272.
HERTZ.—*Brit. Med. Jour.* 1908, i. p. 191.
JACOBI.—*Arch. f. Exp. Path.* 1890.
MACEWEN.—*Lancet*, 1904, ii. 997.

Chapter III

MORBID PHYSIOLOGY OF THE COLON

THE RESULTS OF OCCLUSION OF THE WHOLE OR PART OF THE COLON.

In many operations upon the colon in which an artificial anus is established or a short-circuiting operation is performed, some portion of the colon is left as a blind pouch or, in a few cases, is entirely occluded. In the operation of ileosigmoidostomy, the entire colon is short-circuited or is disconnected from the ileum. There have been many conflicting opinions and much contradictory evidence as to the results that occur in such cases, and the safety to the patient or otherwise in leaving such conditions. I propose here to attempt to consider what changes take place in the colon as the result of such operations.

Senn was one of the first to investigate this subject experimentally. He found that if a portion of the bowel was entirely occluded and its ends closed, it became in time distended, and a source of danger from the accumulation of secretion within it.

Druebert performed iliosigmoidostomy upon dogs and found that, for some weeks after operation, the stools were fluid and the excluded colon remained empty, but after a time the stools became more solid, and fæcal material began to pass backwards into the excluded colon and to accumulate there.

Köste, in a case in which he had excised the cæcum for hyperplastic tuberculosis and implanted the end of the ileum into the sigmoid flexure, narrowed the colon just above the point at which the ileum joined it by means of a ligature, with the object of preventing regurgitation of fæcal material into the colon. In this case there was a fistula communicating with the blind end of the ascending colon, and for six and a half months after operation no fæcal material escaped from the fistula. After this, however, fæces began to come away from the fistula. Köste later divided the splenic flexure and closed the ends. After this, the discharge from the fistula stopped.

Wiessinger found that, out of four cases in which a portion of the colon had been entirely occluded, rupture of the occluded portion or the formation of a fistula occurred in three. Brown occluded a portion of the colon in dogs, and found that, in three to four weeks, the occluded portion was much distended with fæcal-like material; in all cases the distention was greatest at the distal end. Reichel concluded from experiments on animals that accumulation in an occluded loop may or may not occur. Obalinski also concluded from experiment that total occlusion is not followed by serious consequences in the colon, but is dangerous in the small intestine.

In a case of colotomy, the bowel below the artificial opening becomes in course of time considerably atrophied. It loses its pouches, and becomes a smooth and comparatively narrow tube.

I have seen a case in which the end of the sigmoid flexure was closed and an artificial anus established some 6 inches higher up, the blind pouch of pelvic colon being left in the abdomen. The artificial anus did not allow of fæces getting into the blind end, but, in the course of about a year, serious accumulation occurred in the blind pouch, causing ulceration and a fistula.

Lance collected 76 cases of bilateral exclusion. In 8 cases in which the operation was done for fæcal fistula, all recovered. In 68 cases where the operation was done for other conditions, no death or bad result followed. As a method of closing a fæcal fistula, he found bilateral exclusion succeeded in all cases except where malignant disease was present.

The Effects of Leaving Blind or Occluded Portions of the Colon after Resection.—If, after resection of any portion of the colon, an anastomosis be made in such a way as to leave a blind pouch, as for instance, if the end of the descending colon is closed and the ascending or transverse colon anastomosed to the sigmoid flexure, accumulation of fæcal material in the blind pouch will occur. If the blind pouch is a distal one, i.e., if normal peristalsis passes into it, the accumulation will be more serious and occur more rapidly than if it be proximal, i.e., if normal peristalsis passes from it (see *Fig.* 14). But even in the latter case, owing probably to the fact that antiperistalsis occurs normally in the colon, at any rate as far as the upper end of the descending colon, considerable accumulation will eventually occur, and, in course of time, perforation of the end of the blind pouch from stercoral ulceration, and the consequent formation of an abscess, will take place.

This also occurs when the end of the divided ileum is implanted into the sigmoid flexure, as in one method of performing ileosigmoidostomy.

Mr. Arbuthnot Lane, who has performed this operation many times, found that after a time accumulation of fæces and gas occurred in the excluded colon and caused unpleasant symptoms which necessitated its removal. He found that even if only the excluded descending colon was left, accumulation in it still occurred after a time, and it had to be resected.

If the colon is entirely excluded by the formation of an artificial anus in the cæcum, the patient will lose a great quantity of

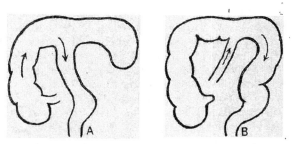

Fig. 14.—Occlusion of the colon by anastomosis with A a distal, and B a proximal blind pouch.

fluid which, under normal circumstances, would be returned into the circulation. When the colon is excluded by ileosigmoidostomy, this loss of fluid is not so marked, owing to the action of the sigmoid in absorbing fluids from the excreta.

Mr. Monier Williams* has recorded a very instructive case in this connection. The patient was a man, aged 52, with ulcerative colitis. An artificial anus was made into the ascending colon close to the cæcum, and a special apparatus was fitted which prevented any of the fæcal material passing into the colon.

The patient improved greatly in health until about a year and a half after the operation, when he began rapidly to lose ground and became emaciated. Half a pint of normal saline solution was then put into the colon daily, and he began to improve

---

* *Brit. Med. Jour.* 1906, i. 787.

again. Three months later, however, he developed purpura hæmorrhagica, and bled profusely. There were several similar attacks, until the plan was adopted of removing the plug in the artificial anus at night and allowing the fæces to pass into the colon, replacing the plug during the day. After this the patient regained perfect health and remained well for three years.

Arbuthnot Lane has found, after resection of the entire colon, that the patients suffer severely from vomiting, which in several cases has threatened to end fatally; this can be prevented by subcutaneous infusion of water.

It is, I think, evident that the loss of body fluids resulting from total exclusion or excision of the colon may seriously interfere with health, and that this loss cannot be entirely compensated by an increased intake of fluid by the mouth. Further, loss of health from that cause may not be evident for a long period after operation. It would seem that it is not the loss of fluid alone, but of some other constituent of the intestinal contents normally absorbed or re-absorbed by the colon, which interferes with the patient's health. In Monier Williams's case, the patient could not be kept in good health by putting water into the colon, but it was necessary to allow the fæces to pass in.

Total excision of the colon has been performed several times by Lane and others, and its loss has been proved to be not incompatible with life or with good health; but we have at present no record of a case showing the condition of the patient two or three years after such an operation.

We may, however, conclude from the foregoing that occlusion of the colon, either partial or total, is a condition which in most cases is not compatible with the permanent maintenance of good health. Accumulation of fæces occurs sooner or later in the occluded loop and causes trouble which, if unrelieved, may give rise to abscess or perforation, and certainly to auto-intoxication.

If the occluded loop is distal to the anastomosis, as in *Fig.* 14 *A*, accumulation will occur rapidly, and if proximal, as in *Fig.* 14 *B*, it will occur more slowly, but it will nevertheless almost certainly take place. Total exclusion of a portion of the colon is not compatible with permanent good health, unless a fistula is left communicating with the excluded portion. If that portion of the colon is left without an external fistulous communication, an abscess will eventually form.

Total excision of the colon is certainly compatible with life; but there is not at present sufficient evidence to show whether or not it is consistent with permanent good health.

Acute Dilatation of the Colon: Meteorism.—Acute dilatation of the colon does not occur apparently as a primary condition, but only as a complication of other diseased states of the bowel. It may occur from interference with the blood-supply of the colon, as in cases of thrombosis of the colic veins, or volvulus of the sigmoid flexure; from inflammation of the peritoneum, as in acute peritonitis; and from obstruction of the lumen of the bowel.

In all cases of thrombosis of the colic veins, acute dilatation of the affected portion of the colon is a marked feature; the dilatation in such cases is not always confined to the portion of colon the blood-supply of which has been injured, for complete obstruction to the passage of fæcal material, and even gas, is caused by the damaged blood-supply, and it is usually found that the bowel, for some distance above the affected area, is also dilated.

The most extreme cases of acute dilatation or meteorism of the colon are those in which the blood-supply is interfered with, when an extraordinary degree of distention of the colon may occur in a few hours. In cases of volvulus of the sigmoid flexure, in which the mesosigmoid is so twisted as to arrest the blood-supply of the sigmoid, great distention of the affected portion of bowel very rapidly occurs. Interference with the venous return of blood from the bowel, the arterial supply remaining intact, would appear to cause a greater degree of distention than total arrest of all the circulation in the colon. It is very difficult to be certain of this point on pure clinical evidence, since it is usually impossible to be certain that the veins alone are blocked in any case of volvulus or other form of strangulation. If we try to compare the cases of thrombosis of the colic veins with cases of pure arterial thrombosis, the cases of the latter condition are so rare that no useful evidence can be brought forward. It is certain, however, that dilatation of the colon occurs in both conditions.

Experimental evidence, however, proves that venous stasis is a more potent factor in causing acute meteorism of the colon than is arterial stasis only. I have performed a number of experiments with the object of ascertaining the causes of dilatation, with the following results:—

THE COLON

If an animal's abdomen is opened and the main veins of a section of the colon are ligatured or clamped, so that the venous flow from that portion of the colon is entirely arrested, and the abdomen is again closed, it will be found in an hour or two, if the abdomen be reopened, that this portion of the colon has become considerably dilated. The affected portion of colon is found to be dusky in colour, and much distended with gas. If some of the gas is removed with a clean glass syringe and tested, it is found to be principally CO_2.

The dilatation occurs very rapidly in spite of the fact that the bowel is open at both ends, as a marked degree of dilatation was present in an hour and a half after the veins had been tied. Clamping or ligature of the arteries going to a similar portion of the colon, produced practically no dilatation in the period covered by the experiment.

It is an easily observed and well known fact, that portions of bowel enclosed within the grasp of intestinal clamps during operations become markedly dilated with gas, even in the short period obtaining during an operation such as lateral anastomosis between portions of the colon, and in gastrojejunostomy.

The CO_2 which accumulates in the bowel and causes the dilatation, results from the fermentative processes occurring in the intestinal contents; the gases (as CO_2 is probably not the only gas present) are normally absorbed by the blood, and carried away in the venous blood-stream under normal conditions; but when the venous stream has been arrested, they accumulate and distend the bowel. When performing the experiments already mentioned, I found that if, before ligating the veins, the colon was first washed out, so that its interior was rendered as clean as possible, no distention with gas occurred.

In performing this experiment, two openings were made at opposite ends of a length of colon, and through them the bowel was washed clean with normal salt solution; the colon was then clamped above and below, so that the cleaned portion was quite isolated, and the openings were then closed. The veins were next all ligated without injury to the arterial supply, and the bowel was returned into the abdomen. At the end of an hour the colon between the clamps was still quite collapsed, and there was no evidence of distention. These experiments were repeated several times, always with the same result. We are therefore, I think, justified in assuming that the gas causing the distention results primarily from fermentative processes in the fæces, and that normally this gas is absorbed by the blood or carried away in the venous blood. The distention is therefore a condition which would normally occur, but is kept in check by the blood-stream under ordinary conditions of health.

These experiments also point out the way in which meteorism may be prevented. It is obvious that this may be done either by emptying the colon, or by introducing some substance which will prevent or delay fermentation.

In order to render these experiments complete, I thought it necessary to prove that the normal mucous membrane of the colon could absorb CO_2. This was done as follows : The ileum of a cat was ligatured just above the ileocæcal valve, and the middle of the colon was similarly ligatured. The upper part of the colon which was thus completely closed was then distended with CO_2 by means of a fine hypodermic needle attached to a gas-bag, the needle being passed obliquely through the bowel wall. The abdomen was then closed. At the end of one hour and forty minutes the occluded portion of colon was examined, when it was found that most of the CO_2 had been absorbed and the bowel was partially collapsed. As the gas could only have escaped by passing through the bowel wall, I think we may assume that it had been carried away in the blood-stream.

Apart from interference with the venous drainage, however, acute dilatation or meteorism of the colon also occurs in cases of acute peritonitis. The most marked dilatation in such cases occurs in the small bowel, but the colon also usually shares in the dilatation, though to a less marked degree. This is no doubt partly due to the fact that the greater area and more central position of the small bowel results in its peritoneal coat being more acutely inflamed than that of the colon in most cases of general peritonitis.

The cause of dilatation in peritonitis is not so obvious as in the conditions previously considered, but it would seem probable that it is due to some interference with the absorbing power of the mucous membrane. The paralysis of the bowel musculature which accompanies acute peritonitis will also obviously be an important factor, because it prevents the fæcal contents being passed on, and enables the latter to accumulate and excessive fermentation to occur ; but arrest of peristalsis will not alone account for the meteorism of peritonitis. When once any marked degree of meteorism has occurred, a "vicious circle" is established : the extreme dilatation of the colon tends to produce kinks and angles in the bowel, which cause obstruction to the lumen ; moreover, the stretching of the bowel wall further paralyzes the muscular walls in the same way that stretching the anal sphincter paralyzes that muscle. It is owing to the establishment of this "vicious circle" that the condition of meteorism, once well established, is so extremely difficult to deal with successfully.

Post-operative Meteorism.—There has at different times been much discussion as to whether post-operative meteorism occurs at all, apart from some degree of peritonitis. It has been noticed that it is more liable to happen in cases where morphia has been administered, and it has been supposed that the morphia was the cause of it. It occurs, however, in cases where no morphia has been given, while it does not take place after abdominal operations performed under the most careful modern surgical technique, where no cause for infection exists, that is, where the bowel has not been opened. I have never seen it, nor been able to find an instance of it, except in cases where there were obvious possibilities of some infection. Also it has become decidedly less common in the last few years, since more careful aseptic methods have prevailed.

These facts, and its close resemblance to meteorism occurring as a symptom of general peritonitis, make it almost certain that it is the result of microbic infection of the peritoneum. It usually occurs within forty-eight hours after an operation, accompanied by pain, raised temperature, and other signs of peritoneal infection, and in those cases where it has proved fatal, signs of peritonitis are present.

In acute dilatation of the colon, the walls of the bowel are thinned and stretched so that in some cases they may be almost transparent. The tension within the bowel may be considerable, and it has happened, on opening the abdomen for the purpose of relieving an obstruction, that the visceral peritoneum covering the distended bowel has split directly the support of the abdominal wall has been removed. It is advisable, when operating in cases of well-marked meteorism, to make as small an abdominal incision as possible, in order to avoid this danger.

When the colon becomes dilated above a stricture or other obstruction of the bowel lumen, the distention occurs much more slowly than in those cases where the blood-supply of the colon has been damaged, or where there is peritonitis.

It is certain that the only satisfactory method of dealing with meteorism is to empty the colon of its contents and thus prevent the fermentation which causes it. This may be done by opening a distended coil and emptying the contents by some such method as that invented by Moynihan, with a long tube on to which successive coils can be pulled.

Chapter IV.

BACTERIOLOGY OF THE COLON.

The number of micro-organisms present in the intestinal contents of man and the mammalia is enormous; it has been estimated that there are on an average one hundred and twenty-six billions for the daily human excreta.

The fact that the digestive tract is so rich in bacteria has led many physiologists to the belief that they are essential to the well-being of the host. Pasteur expressed this view, and other observers, such as Schottelius, Madame Metchnikoff, and Moro, have agreed with him, and experiments in which chickens, tadpoles, and turtle larvæ have been fed on sterile food, with the result that their development was retarded, are brought forward in support of this view.

These experiments are not, however, conclusive; on the other hand, Nuttall and Thierpelder reared guinea-pigs, delivered by Cæsarean section, on sterile food, and the animals lived and increased in weight. More important are the observations of Levin, that many of the animals in the Arctic regions have no bacteria in their digestive tract. He investigated the intestinal contents of Arctic animals at Spitzbergen, and found that, in most instances, in white bears, seals, reindeer, eider-ducks, and penguins, the digestive tracts were entirely sterile. This, I think, proves conclusively that bacteria in the intestinal tract are not in any way necessary to life, and it is probably correct to look upon their presence rather as a necessary feature of residence in warm or temperate climates, and, like dirt and bacteria upon the surface of the body, as being to a large extent unavoidable.

It is probable, however, that in the case of mammals whose digestive tract usually contains large numbers of micro-organisms, certain types of bacteria which are normally found in great numbers in the intestinal contents are actually of value to the animal in keeping down and suppressing the growth of other and more harmful bacteria which may from time to time obtain an entrance. The best instance of this is seen in the case of *B. coli*. Immense numbers of *B. coli* are normally present in the human intestine, and experiments show that they tend to hinder the development of putrefactive decomposition of the intestinal contents, and also to combat the growth of injurious saprophytes usually present. Thus fluids liable to undergo rapid putrefaction may be kept for days or even weeks without change if they contain large quantities of *B. coli*, even though *B. putrificans* be added ; whereas, if *B. coli* be not present, putrefaction will occur rapidly.

The Distribution of Bacteria in the Intestinal Tract.—The greatest number of bacteria are found in the large intestine. In dogs the large intestine is closely crowded with bacteria just beyond the ileocæcal valve, whatever may be the conditions of the ileum. The living bacteria, however, steadily decrease in number as we pass down the colon, so that in the rectum they are much less numerous than in the ascending colon and cæcum.

There is some reason to suppose that in certain cases of disease of the colon what may be called the " phenomenon of substitution of one type of bacteria for another " occurs. In other words, the colon bacillus, which is the normal dominant organism of the large intestine, becomes replaced by another form of organism which, though normally present, exists only in small numbers under conditions of health. Thus Herter quotes the case of a woman suffering from colitis, in whom the dominant *B. coli* disappeared and was replaced by a different organism, but with restoration to health the *B. coli* again became the dominant organism.

Lactic Acid Bacilli.—Recently this phenomenon of substitution has been taken advantage of as a means of treating certain infective diseases of the colon. Prof. Metchnikoff was the first to point out the principles of treating certain diseases of the colon by the administration of curdled milk, and his methods have since been elaborated by several other workers, notably by Cohendy working at the Pasteur Institute, and Herschell in this country.* The principle of the treatment consists in giving by the mouth large quantities of the Bulgarian lactic acid bacillus, either in pure culture or in the form of soured

---

* "Soured milk and pure cultures of lactic acid bacilli in the treatment of disease " (G. Herschell).

milk. This bacillus is able to escape the action of the gastric juices, and on reaching the colon it inhibits the growth of proteolytic microbes which it finds there, and even destroys them. The effect of its introduction is to enormously reduce the number of other bacteria in the stools, and even occasionally to entirely get rid of them. The lactic acid bacteria, in fact, are substituted for the ordinary microbes present in the colon, and as they are quite harmless to the host, we are thus enabled to replace harmful organisms in the colon by others which we know to be harmless.

The Bulgarian bacillus occurs normally in the human fæces, but only in small quantities. It is a large bacillus, which stains easily by the usual methods and is Gram-positive. It may be cultivated in milk, in milk serum to which 1·5 of peptone has been added, and upon milk peptone agar. On the latter it grows in round whitish colonies. It can be administered by the mouth, either as soured milk, or as liquid or dried cultures. After it has been administered for a short time it replaces the putrefactive bacteria in the colon, and may be found in the fæces in almost pure culture. It has been much used in the treatment of autointoxication, a condition in which there is sometimes excessive bacterial growth in the colon. It inhibits the growth of *Bacillus coli*, and may therefore be used in cases where we suspect this organism of causing disease.

Experiment showing Conditions of Anaerobic Growth in the Intestine of the Dog (Herter).—Dog weighing 14½ lbs. The dog was given 200 mgrams of methylene blue in water. On the third day he was given 100 mgrams of methylene blue in a piece of cooked meat. Four hours after eating the meat he was killed and the intestine examined. The stomach was

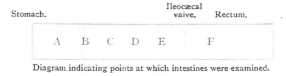

Diagram indicating points at which intestines were examined.

intensely blue. The duodenum was blue, but the intensity of the colour diminished towards B ; at C the colour had almost disappeared, while it had entirely gone between C and D. The contents of the intestine at D only became blue on exposure to air. The contents of the intestine between E and F were not blue until exposed to air.

This experiment indicates that beyond the middle of the small intestine the conditions become rapidly anaerobic, since the reduction of methylene blue could not occur in the presence of air in this concentration.

Bacillus coli.—The question as to whether the *B. coli* can become virulent and cause pathological processes within the colon is a difficult one. (I am leaving out of account for the present any pathological processes which may result from *B. coli* that have reached other tissues—as by perforation of the bowel wall, etc.)

The subject is the more difficult as, in most cases in which it would appear that a pathological process has been set up in the colon by *B. coli*, the organism has not been properly identified, and many other intestinal organisms closely resemble the *B. coli*, and cannot be distinguished from them except by careful biochemical tests. It seems probable that *B. coli* cannot initiate putrefactive processes in the colon, but if putrefactive anaerobes be present, the *B. coli* can take an active part in breaking down hydrolysed proteids.

Tubercle Bacilli.—In cases of intestinal tuberculosis, and especially if ulcerative lesions of the alimentary tract are present, it is usual for tubercle bacilli to be found in the stools, and these may readily be demonstrated by suitable methods.

Owing, however, to the large number of organisms usually present in fæces, it is necessary that a very careful examination be made to prevent the possibility of confusing other and similar organisms for the tubercle bacillus. Quite apart, however, from intestinal tuberculosis, it is not uncommon to find the tubercle bacillus in fæces. Rosenberger, with a view of determining how frequently tubercle bacilli are present in fæces, examined the stools of 672 patients in the wards of the Philadelphia General Hospital. The cases examined included pneumonia, typhoid, erysipelas, diarrhœa, and numerous other conditions, both medical and surgical, and some apparently healthy patients. In sixty of the cases some form of tuberculous lesion was known to be present. In all these 60 cases tubercle bacilli were present in the fæces, while in 120 of the other cases, or in 19·6 per cent, tubercle bacilli were found in the stools.

From this it is obvious that too much significance must not be attached to the presence of acid-fast bacilli in the stools, and that they may be present without any intestinal tuberculous lesion.

Chapter V.

METHODS OF DIAGNOSIS.

The colon is a very inaccessible portion of the human body, and when the site of disease is unknown it is not easy correctly to diagnose the condition or to ascertain the position and nature of the lesion. There are, however, at the present day, several means at our disposal by which we can obtain exact and reliable data to aid us in accurately diagnosing the cause of the symptoms and the situation of the lesion. It is often necessary to employ several or all of these in the same case, to carefully compare the results, and examine them in reference to the symptoms and history, before attempting to make a diagnosis.

In any difficult case it is seldom either possible or advisable to attempt a diagnosis as to the condition present in the colon from a single examination, and several days are often necessary to complete a thorough investigation.

Until quite recently, disease of the colon was generally diagnosed from the symptoms, but whenever possible, we should base our conclusions upon facts rather than symptoms, as the latter, especially in the case of the colon, are extremely unreliable and misleading.

History and Symptoms.—The patient's past history, as well as the history of the symptoms, should be most carefully gone into.

If there is pain, it is necessary to ascertain the time at which it comes on, its duration, severity, whether relieved by lying down or stooping, its position, and so on. The history of the present symptoms should be enquired into, and any history of previous abdominal or bowel trouble is most important, such as appendicitis, peritonitis, gastric ulcer, etc.

The condition of the stools should be enquired into : whether there is blood or discharge ; if there is mucus, and whether in the form of shreds, slime, or casts. Their colour and consistence, whether solid or liquid, are all important points. If there is diarrhœa, it is important to know whether much or little is passed at a time, how many stools there are in twenty-four hours, whether there is tenesmus, the time of day at which the stools are most frequent, and especially whether there is a desire to go to stool on first rising in the morning.

If there is constipation, we must ask whether aperients are taken, and if so, in what quantities, and how often; also whether there are periods of diarrhœa. We should ask whether the patient has lost weight; if so, how much, and in what time. It must, however, be remembered that diarrhœa, if it has persisted for some time, almost invariably results in loss of weight.

Many patients who suffer from bowel troubles are very neurotic, and inclined to attach unnecessary importance to their symptoms and to exaggerate them. For this reason it is advisable to obtain some estimate of the amount of pain, discomfort, and other symptoms which depend upon the patient's sensations, by asking about the details of his daily life. Thus, if the patient complains of severe abdominal pain, we can often gauge its severity by ascertaining whether he has to go to bed, whether it interferes with his occupation, and if it prevents his sleeping.

It is important to go carefully into the history of the case, as by so doing we gain the patient's confidence, and at the same time form a valuable estimate of the gravity of the condition, and get an indication as to the probable cause of the trouble; but it is the greatest mistake to attempt a diagnosis from the history and symptoms alone. Such a diagnosis is more than likely to be wrong; the history and symptoms are frequently most misleading, and it is better not to allow ourselves to be biassed towards any particular diagnosis until a thorough examination has been made. After the results of this are known, the history of the case should be carefully studied with the object of explaining the findings, and for confirmatory evidence. In fact, the examination should form the ground-work for the diagnosis, and the history and symptoms should be considered secondary. Too often the diagnosis is built up the other way, and facts are made to fit the evidence, whereas the evidence should only be used to confirm and supplement the facts.

General Inspection.—We should notice whether the patient is fat or thin, and if the latter, whether there is emaciation. The presence of anæmia or cachexia may also be noticed. The

METHODS OF DIAGNOSIS

condition of the abdomen is important, especially as to whether it is flat or distended, whether the abdominal wall is firm, flabby or pendulous. The presence or absence of hernia should always be noted. The patient should be examined standing up with the abdomen exposed, to ascertain whether there is any bulging of the lower abdomen, as is often the case in visceroptosis.

Palpation of the Abdomen.—For this purpose the patient must be placed in the correct position. The head and shoulders should be supported on a pillow, and the knees should be well drawn up, so that the feet rest flat on the couch and do not tend to slip down. The patient is told not to talk, and to allow the abdomen to be as loose as possible. The whole abdomen must be carefully palpated. Any tender spots should be noted, and whether the tenderness is deep or superficial.

The colon, if normal, cannot be felt, but in many abnormal conditions it can be distinctly felt, especially on the left side. Of course, if the sigmoid is loaded with fæces, it can easily be felt, and it is always advisable, when possible, to examine the abdomen again after the bowels have been well cleared with aperients or enemata. Tumours may be felt after the bowels have been well emptied, which were quite impalpable previously.

Additional information may sometimes be obtained by placing the patient in different positions, as for instance on the side, and in the knee-elbow position.

Before leaving the examination of the abdomen, the stomach should be mapped out by percussion, as its lower border is a useful guide to the position of the transverse colon. Both this and the lower border of the liver should be marked while the patient is lying down, and then with the patient standing they should be marked out again, when if visceroptosis is present there will be a considerable difference in the two positions.

As an aid to percussion, the bowel may in some cases be gently inflated with air introduced per anum, after the bowel has been emptied. This will enable us to ascertain—often with considerable accuracy—the position of the sigmoid flexure and transverse colon.

This method of inflating the bowel requires to be employed with considerable caution, and on no account should air be forcibly introduced into the bowel, as I have seen recommended. The bowel may easily be ruptured by forcible distention, and considerable pain will certainly be caused. The method I prefer is to place the patient in the knee-elbow position and pass a rectal tube. This allows air to pass into the empty colon under normal atmospheric pressure, and if then the tube is removed, and the patient examined in the recumbent position, the sigmoid can usually be readily mapped out.

If the examination is to be completed at one sitting, it is advisable to postpone the palpation of the abdomen until after the sigmoidoscope has been used, otherwise the examination of the abdomen may force fæcal matter down into the sigmoid, and thus interfere with the use of the instrument.

SIGMOIDOSCOPY.

This is perhaps the most valuable means we have of examining the colon, and should never be omitted. It is true that with the

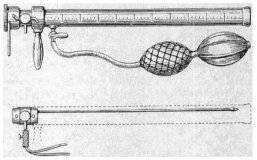

Fig. 15.—Author's modification of Strauss's sigmoidoscope.

sigmoidoscope we can only examine the pelvic portion of the colon, and this is only a small part of the whole; but on the other hand, this is the part most commonly diseased, and when other parts of the colon are diseased, the pelvic portion also is generally involved.

There are several different patterns of sigmoidoscope, but by far the best is that originally designed by Professor Strauss. The author has, however, slightly modified the original instrument (*Fig.* 15), and has substituted metal filament lamps, which only require two or four volts, for the original carbon ones. These lamps give a better light and do not get hot, while they have the additional advantage of working off a small battery, which is easily portable.

SIGMOIDOSCOPY

The chief difficulty in making a satisfactory examination is to get the sigmoid flexure empty. It is only when very skilfully administered that the entire sigmoid can be emptied by enemata. The best plan is to give a rhubarb or colocynth pill twenty-four hours before the examination, followed by a plain warm-water

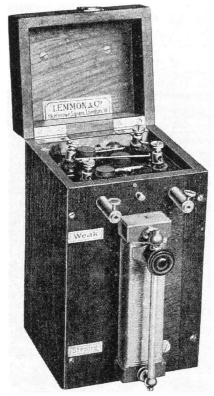

Fig. 16.—A portable accumulator fitted with a rheostat for working the sigmoidoscope.

enema some three or four hours before the examination. In cases of ulcerative colitis or stricture, it is better to omit the aperient and use only the enema.

If properly manipulated, the instrument does not cause pain or serious discomfort, and an anæsthetic is not necessary, though it is sometimes advisable.

SIGMOIDOSCOPY

The patient may be examined either in the knee-elbow position, or in the left Sims' or semi-prone position. The former is the easier position for the surgeon (*Fig.* 17), the latter the most comfortable for the patient. If the semi-prone position be adopted, a small, hard cushion should be placed under the left hip, the knees should be well drawn up, and the feet placed well forward, so as to be out of the way of the surgeon (*Fig.* 18). The examination is best made with the patient on a high couch or operating-table.

Method of Passing the Tube.—Before introducing the tube, the portion carrying the lamp is withdrawn and the obturator

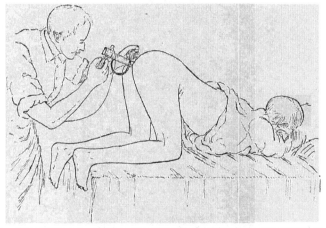

Fig. 17.—Sigmoidoscopic examination of the colon with the patient in the genu-pectoral position.

inserted. The instrument should then be warmed by pouring some hot water over it. This is better than dipping into hot water, as the inside of the tube is not made wet. The tube should then be well smeared over with vaseline, and some vaseline put on the anus. The instrument should be carefully inserted into the anus, and pushed gently onwards till it has entered about four inches; the end of the instrument should be kept in a backward direction toward the sacrum. As soon as it has gone in this distance the obturator should be removed, and the lamp portion of the tube inserted in its place. The switch can now be turned on, and a little air pumped into the bowel by means of

SIGMOIDOSCOPY

the rubber bellows. The tube should now be passed gently onwards by sight. The surgeon should look for the lumen of the bowel, and gently insinuate the end of the tube into it, if necessary pumping in a little air to open out the bowel walls. All manipulations should be as gentle as possible. The end of the instrument must not be pressed against the mucous membrane, but the folds of the bowel pushed aside by a slight puff of air. In this way the instrument is passed by sight, and the end of the tube need not even touch the mucous membrane,

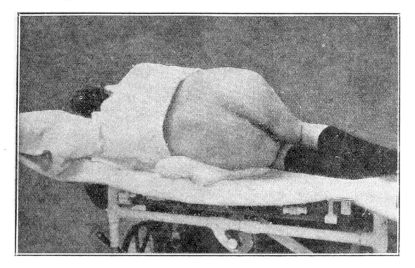

Fig. 18.—The Sims' position for passing the sigmoidoscope.

but work its way behind a cushion of air. Thus there is no danger of causing damage to the walls of the bowel, however diseased they may be. It is necessary, in order to ensure success, that the direction of the bowel, when tracing it up from the anus, should be remembered. At first the bowel passes backwards, following the curve of the sacrum, then it turns very sharply forward to pass over the sacral prominence, and in order to get the end of the tube over this prominence it must be carried forward.

At the junction of the rectum with the sigmoid there is always a well-developed fold of mucous membrane similar to the valves of Houston. This partly occludes the bowel lumen, and, being situated anteriorly, the end of the instrument is very liable to be caught by it as it is being carried forward over the sacral prominence. It is partly this valve, and partly the sharp bend of the bowel which usually occurs here, that makes it difficult to pass the instrument into the sigmoid flexure. As a rule, the sigmoid passes to the left just after the recto-sigmoidal junction, but this is not invariable, and it may be found to pass to the right or straight forward in exceptional cases.

As has been stated, considerable difficulty may be experienced in getting the instrument to enter the sigmoid. The upper portion of the rectum below the recto-sigmoidal junction is very capacious, and often forms a sort of cul-de-sac behind this junction; or, at any rate, there appears to be such a cul-de-sac in certain cases. What happens is that, after the tube has passed over the sacral prominence, the bowel appears to end blindly, no continuation of the lumen being observable. In such cases the opening into the sigmoid will usually be found situated lower down and anteriorly.

When the end of the tube has entered the sigmoid flexure, it usually has to be deflected rather towards the patient's left side, though, as has already been stated, it may have to be passed to the right side in exceptional cases. The tube is a straight one, and, of course, cannot go round curves; but what really happens is that the sigmoid flexure, which is a freely movable portion of the bowel, is threaded on to the instrument much in the same way as the finger of a glove is drawn on a stick.

Care must be used in negotiating sharp curves, and on no account must the instrument be forced round the curve if there is definite resistance. The use of force under such circumstances causes pain by putting the mesentery on the stretch, and might even tear it. With practice, there is usually little difficulty in passing the instrument to its full length. The changes in the direction of the tube while being passed are shown roughly in the diagram (*Fig.* 19).

After the tube has been introduced as far as it will go, it is slowly withdrawn, during which operation the whole lumen of the bowel comes into view, and any growth, ulceration, or other abnormality present can be detected and examined. Should a growth be found, its exact dimensions can easily be ascertained, and by watching whether or not it moves with the intestinal wall on inflating the bowel, or by pushing it gently with the end of the tube, one can easily determine its mobility and estimate

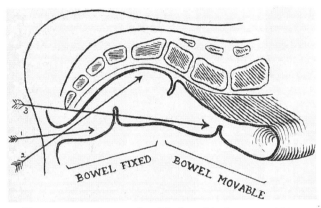

Fig. 19.—Diagram to show the successive deflections of the instrument which are necessary in the process of introduction. The arrows show the direction of the tube at each point. The bend of the bowel to the left at the recto-sigmoidal junction is indicated, together with the approximate positions of the valves of Houston.

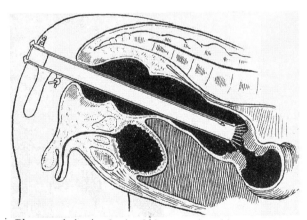

Fig. 20.—Diagrammatic drawing showing the instrument in position for examining a growth at the lower end of the sigmoid flexure.

the chances of successfully removing it by operation. The distance of any lesion from the anus is ascertained by looking at the graduated scale on the outside of the tube. Should it be necessary to swab away any blood or fæcal material from the surface of the growth, or even to remove portions of it for microscopical examination, this can be done by removing the back glass of the instrument and passing swabs on special holders down the tube, or by using special forceps made for the purpose.

The distance to which the instrument can be passed varies considerably with different patients. In those who have a long sigmoid mesentery and no adhesions round the bowel, it is usually possible to pass the instrument to its full length, and to see well beyond the middle of the sigmoid flexure. When, however, the mesentery is short, or the bowel is surrounded by adhesions, it cannot be passed beyond the last loop of the sigmoid.

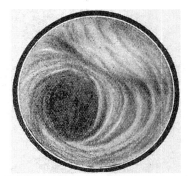

Fig. 21.—Left internal iliac artery seen through the wall of the sigmoid flexure.

The instrument is not so easily passed in women as in men, chiefly owing to the fact that the angle of the sacrum is much greater in women, and consequently the rectum has a greater curve.

I have had considerable experience with this instrument, and have never met with any unpleasant results from its use. Instances have occurred in which the bowel has been damaged, but this has only happened to inexperienced operators, and has been due to the use of force when introducing the tube. Under no circumstances should any force be used, and once it has entered the rectum it should be passed entirely by sight.

One little warning in connection with the use of the sigmoidoscope is worth giving. If during the examination it is

necessary to remove the lamp attachment, or to open the back of the tube by removal of the glass window—as, for instance, when a swab-holder or other instrument is to be passed down the tube—the air should be allowed to escape slowly, either by the tap or by opening the glass window slowly. If this is suddenly removed, and there is any pressure of air in the bowel, the bowel wall may be pushed into the end of the tube when the pressure is released, and the mucous membrane be injured.
. I have found that there is seldom any necessity to pump in much air ; all that is required is an occasional puff to straighten the bowel. If a quantity is introduced it induces peristalsis, which defeats the surgeon's object, and causes the patient discomfort.

The condition of the mucous membrane of the pelvic colon should be carefully examined, also the mobility of this portion of the colon. The normal sigmoid flexure is quite freely movable in all directions, and if, except at its junction with the rectum, it is found to be fixed and cannot be moved from one position, we may assume the presence of adhesions or a tumour, though there is the possibility of a very short mesocolon.

Those readers who wish to learn to use the instrument are advised to read *The Sigmoidoscope*, by the same author.

THE USE OF X RAYS
IN THE DIAGNOSIS OF DISEASE OF THE COLON.

In obscure cases, valuable information is sometimes obtained by the aid of X-ray examinations. The method is somewhat difficult, and requires the very best apparatus ; small installations will not give sufficient penetration. This method is particularly useful in cases of ptosis or displacement of the colon, and has also been employed in the diagnosis of strictures. In cases of constipation it may be used to ascertain in which portion of the colon the delay occurs. Dr. Hertz, who devised this method of examining cases of constipation, has by means of it made valuable observations in such cases.

In order that the colon may throw a shadow, it is necessary that it should contain some substance which will arrest the rays. For this purpose bismuth, suspended in a liquid or semi-liquid vehicle, is usually employed. The bismuth may either be given by the mouth with food, or injected through the anus directly into the colon. The method adopted depends upon the circumstances of the case. When we wish to ascertain either the position of the sigmoid flexure, or if there is a stricture, it is better to inject the bismuth directly into the colon. It is probably also the better method in cases of ptosis of the transverse colon. When, however, we wish to examine the progress of a test meal through the colon, the bismuth should be given by the mouth.

In adopting the latter plan the method is as follows :—

The patient is given a breakfast consisting of bread and milk, with which two ounces of bismuth carbonate have been well mixed. The bismuth will reach the cæcum in a normal individual in a little over four hours, and after this the patient must be examined periodically with the X rays. The patient is laid flat on his back on a couch, with the X-ray tube beneath the couch and under the centre of the abdomen. A coin should be placed on the umbilicus, as it affords a useful landmark. The screen is placed across the abdomen, and on this is laid a piece of thin tissue paper. The outline of the shadow is then traced on the tissue paper, and marks made to indicate the positions of the umbilicus and anterior superior spines; the time of the examination should also be marked on the paper. A series of examinations are made, and afterwards, by comparing the tracings, the point at which delay, if any, occurred in the passage of the bismuth, and any abnormalities in the position of the different portions of the colon, can be seen. It is not correct, however, to assume, because we find the bismuth unduly delayed in its passage, through the ascending colon for instance, that therefore the cause of its delay is at the hepatic flexure. It may equally well be in the sigmoid flexure, the bismuth being arrested because the bowel contents in front of it cannot pass on. The negative evidence is valuable, however, as, for instance, if we find that the bismuth has passed in about the normal time through the colon until it reaches the sigmoid flexure, we are safe in assuming that there is no obstruction in the rest of the colon (see *Fig.* 12).

The normal times for the bismuth to reach different parts of the colon are given by Hertz as follows : To reach the cæcum $4\frac{1}{2}$ hours, hepatic flexure $6\frac{1}{2}$ hours, splenic flexure 9 hours, sigmoid flexure about 12 hours.

These figures are only approximate; considerable variations may occur, and during sleep the progress is much slower.

Where the bismuth is to be introduced directly into the colon,

PLATE II

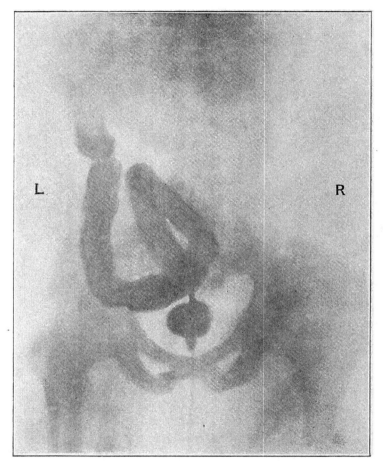

RADIOGRAPH OF THE PELVIC COLON after the injection of bismuth emulsion, showing a cancerous stricture at the recto-sigmoidal junction.
(OKINCZYC, *Cancer du Côlon*: Steinheil, Paris.)

OF DISEASES OF THE COLON 53

it should be made into a thick emulsion with olive oil; the quantity required is from 200 to 400 cc.

The patient is placed in the genu-pectoral position during the introduction of the emulsion, and a long rectal tube is passed into the sigmoid flexure by means of the sigmoidoscope, the instrument being afterwards withdrawn over the tube so as to leave the latter in place. Unless the tube is passed through the sigmoidoscope it is impossible to be certain that it is in the

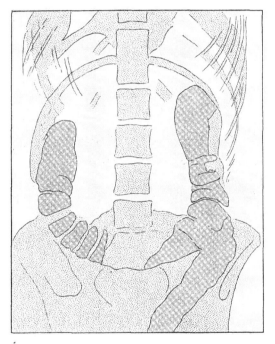

Fig. 22.—X ray photograph of a patient after bismuth emulsion has been injected into the colon. The photograph shows extensive prolapse of the tranverse colon—visceroptosis.
(*After Schule, from La Presse Médicale.*)

sigmoid. By injecting the emulsion through the tube we avoid distending the rectal ampulla and so causing tenesmus, the presence of the emulsion is more easily tolerated, and a larger quantity can be introduced. By placing the patient in the genu-pectoral position the emulsion is enabled to pass up into the higher parts of the colon.

54 THE USE OF X RAYS IN DIAGNOSIS

If the patient is unable to remain long enough in this position, the injection should be given in the left Sims' position, and the foot of the couch well raised on blocks. The X-ray examination is made in the same way. The bismuth seems to be well tolerated by the bowel, and does not cause any unpleasant consequences as a rule. A stricture in the bowel is generally indicated by a dense shadow above and below it, but deceptive

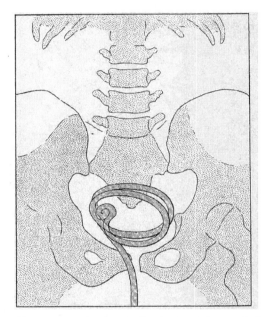

Fig. 23.—X-ray photograph of a patient after the introduction of a long rectal tube. Note that the tube has curled up in the rectum and not entered the colon.
(*After Schule, from La Presse Médicale.*)

appearances are liable to occur. These methods of X-ray diagnosis in disease or abnormalities of the colon are comparatively new, and are only of use in certain cases. The results so obtained must not be too implicitly relied on, but used rather as confirmatory evidence.

The X rays are of the greatest value in localizing foreign bodies in the colon, and may also assist in the detection of stercoliths.

Diagnosis by Means of Rectal Bougies and Tubes.—The use of rectal bougies for the diagnosis of strictures in the bowel was at one time very popular, but they have now been entirely replaced by the sigmoidoscope and similar instruments. It is well that it is so, for the use of bougies is by no means free from danger, and there have been numerous accidents due to perforation of the bowel wall; moreover, they are of very little value in diagnosis, as the end may easily be arrested by one of the rectal valves, and so give the impression that a stricture exists, when as a matter of fact there is none.

Diagnoses based on the passage of a rectal tube are quite valueless. One not uncommonly hears it stated that a patient in whose colon the presence of a stricture is suspected, has no stricture in the sigmoid flexure, because a rectal tube has easily been passed for two feet. This, however, proves nothing, as the tube usually curls up in the rectum, and although two feet of it have been introduced, the end may lie just within the anus. Any one who doubts this statement has only to examine the patient with X rays, after passing the tube, to be convinced; they will see the tube coiled up in the rectal ampulla (*Fig. 23*).

The only way in which a long tube can with certainty be introduced into the colon is by passing it through the sigmoidoscope.

It is very doubtful whether a tube can be passed up the bowel for more than six inches once in twenty times, and the so-called high enemas given with a long tube could be just as well administered with an enema nozzle.

Examination Under an Anæsthetic.—This is a most valuable aid to diagnosis in difficult cases. With the abdominal muscles well relaxed, the whole colon can be palpated, and if a tumour is present it can usually be felt. A bimanual examination should also be made with two fingers in the rectum. If the sphincters are slightly stretched, the two first fingers of the right hand can easily be passed into the bowel, and this allows one to reach nearly an inch higher than if only one finger is employed. By bimanual examination, growths in the lower third of the sigmoid can usually be felt through the anterior rectal wall. Abscesses in the iliac fossæ can also be felt, and the pelvic organs explored.

The examination should first be made with the patient lying on his back, and he should then be turned over on his side, and the knees well drawn up. The examination should then be repeated. The change in attitude may allow a tumour to fall forward into a position in which it can be more easily felt; also, when a tumour has already been detected, valuable information as to its mobility or otherwise is afforded by palpation with the patient in different positions.

Exploratory Laparotomy.—This should not often be necessary, and if the patient has been carefully examined by the means already mentioned, an approximate diagnosis will, at any rate, have been arrived at in most cases. Exploratory laparotomy should never be performed unless there are reasonable grounds for supposing that a lesion exists which can only be treated satisfactorily by operation, and it should not be used merely as a method of diagnosis. Before deciding upon such an operation, a consultation is advisable, and the question of whether the results likely to accrue from the operation are commensurate with the risks, will have to be carefully considered.

There are cases, however, where there is good reason to assume that some lesion in the colon exists which may be easily remedied by an operation, but the exact situation, or even its actual presence, cannot be determined with any certainty; in such cases, after due consideration, exploratory laparotomy is unquestionably indicated.

Examination of the Stools.—This is always an important factor in diagnosis, which should never be omitted. The shape and character of the deposits should be noted. Liquid stools, except when aperients are taken, are always a sign of something abnormal. Constant fluid fæces, mixed with jelly-like mucus, generally result from a stricture or ulceration in the bowel.

Much importance is often attached to the shape of the fæces when solid. Thus it is stated that ribbon-like or "pipe-stem" fæces indicate a stricture or narrowing in the bowel. This is a most fallacious argument. Though it is true that if a stricture exists at the anal opening the fæces may be flattened or otherwise altered in shape, a stricture higher up in the bowel cannot affect the shape of the fæces, as the mass would inevitably be reformed in the rectal ampulla and must take its shape from the last narrow opening through which it passes—the anus.

The shape and form of the fæces are of little, if any, diagnostic value.

The presence of abnormal constituents is important. Mucus

OF DISEASES OF THE COLON

is normally present in the stools, but not in sufficient quantity to be obvious. The presence of large quantities of mucus is indicative of some irritative lesion. Much importance is often attached to the form in which the mucus is found, whether it be in that of slime, shreds, or casts. It is doubtful, however, whether we can attach any significance to its form. A patient will at one time pass jelly-like mucus and at another well-formed casts or membranes. I have seen large casts passed by patients who were suffering from cancer of the sigmoid. The exact reason for the mucus forming casts in some cases and not in others is not understood, and we are not justified in drawing any conclusions from their presence (*vide* Chapter II.).

Blood.—The presence of blood in the stools is of great importance, as it indicates the presence of ulceration or some breach of surface—with the rare exception of some of the hæmophylic conditions. Blood may often be present in such small quantity that it is not obvious to the naked eye, and some test for its presence is necessary. There are several chemical tests for blood in the stools, but a microscopical examination of the fæces affords the best and most reliable.

About an ounce of liquid stool should be collected in a clean bottle, and to this about the same quantity of 5 per cent formalin solution added. A microscopical examination demonstrates the presence of blood, undigested food, or parasites, and may enable us to detect portions of malignant growth.

Urine.—A careful examination of the urine is often valuable, as by this means we may ascertain whether autointoxication is occurring. The presence of indican in the urine, or indicanuria, shows that excessive albuminous putrefaction is occurring somewhere in the body. Its presence is very often a sign of intestinal putrefaction, and its quantity varies with the activity of that process. It is invariably present in cases of severe constipation in which there is autointoxication.

Obermeyer's test for indican in the urine is as follows : Take 50 cc. of urine, add to it 10 cc. of a 20 per cent solution of lead acetate ; then filter. The filtrate must be well shaken with an equal quantity of hydrochloric acid containing between 0·2 and 0·4 per cent ferric chloride, and a few cubic centimetres of chloroform. If indican is present in the urine, indigo-blue will be formed, and will pass into solution in the chloroform.

Chapter VI.

CONGENITAL ABNORMALITIES OF THE COLON.

CONGENITAL abnormalities of the colon may be conveniently divided into: Congenital abnormalities of the colon itself: and Congenital abnormalities of the peritoneum or mesentery.

CONGENITAL ABNORMALITIES OF THE COLON ITSELF.

These are very rare, and as a rule, when present, are found to be associated with congenital abnormalities in other parts.

The colon, or some part of it, may be completely absent, or represented only by a fibrous cord. Some form of atresia is the commonest condition met with. Thus, some portion of the colon may be represented only by a narrow tube. In Atkins' case the whole colon and rectum were rudimentary, and about the thickness of an ordinary quill, there being a small lumen, however, throughout the colon. The condition in this case was associated with imperforate anus.

In another case, the ascending and transverse portions of the colon were represented by a narrow tube about the thickness of a lead pencil, while the remainder was normal, except for some annular contractions in the sigmoid. The condition in this case was associated with an hour-glass contraction of the stomach, and a stricture of the ileum just above the ileocæcal valve, also of congenital origin.

A very interesting case was recorded by Anderson, of an infant who was born with a fæcal fistula at the umbilicus and an imperforate anus. Post mortem it was found that the fæcal fistula was formed by the ileum immediately above the ileocæcal valve being adherent to the umbilicus. The cæcum, ascending, transverse, and descending portions of the colon were present, but the descending colon ended in a blind extremity. There was no trace of any sigmoid flexure or rectum.

CONGENITAL ABNORMALITIES

A case is recorded by Lockwood, in which the descending colon was double. The two tubes were parallel with each other, and both were provided with a lumen and appendices epiploicæ; one was, however, very small, while the other was of fair diameter and performed the functions of the descending colon. The patient was a man, aged 57, who died at St. Bartholomew's Hospital from intestinal obstruction. There was a malignant growth at the lower end of the descending colon at the spot at which the two tubes appeared to join again.

Congenital stenosis of the colon is very rare, but there are several cases on record. The stenosis may consist of a diaphragm or may take a tubular form. In a few instances more than one stricture has been present.

CONGENITAL ABNORMALITIES OF THE PERITONEUM OR MESENTERY.

The commonest congenital abnormalities of the colon are those in which there has been some failure in the descent of the cæcum, or rather where the normal development of the peritoneal connections of the colon has been arrested. It is obvious, from a study of the development of the colon in relation to its peritoneal attachments, that any abnormality may exist, between the colon being represented by a practically straight tube and the normal condition.

If arrest of development takes place at a very early date, the cæcum will be outside the abdomen, and the colon be represented by a practically straight tube between the umbilicus and the rectum.

The cæcum may be situated in the left side of the abdomen (quite apart from complete transposition of the viscera). This may occur in two ways: (1) From arrested development at an early stage before the cæcum has passed across to the right hypochondrium, or (2) From persistence of the cæcal mesentery allowing the cæcum to migrate to the left side.

In Professor Simpson's case the cæcum was retained in an umbilical hernia by adhesions, the result of intra-uterine inflammation, and the colon retained the primitive form of a straight tube. There is a specimen of a similar case in the museum of the Royal College of Surgeons.

The cæcum may be found on the left side of the abdomen near the spleen, and the transverse colon be absent. Several such cases have been recorded, and in most of them it is stated that the cæcum was fixed by adhesions. It seems probable that the original lesion was an abnormal mesentery to the cæcum, which allowed it to migrate to the left side of the abdomen, where it became fixed by adhesions.

A more common condition is for the cæcum to fail to descend into the right iliac fossa, and to remain just beneath the liver. This condition is normally present in many mammals. In such cases the ascending colon is unrepresented, and the cæcum communicates directly with the transverse colon. In the male the non-descent of the cæcum is often associated with imperfect descent of the right testicle.

A very curious case was reported by Elliott Smith, in which the cæcum, as such, appeared to be absent. The ileum passed insensibly into the ascending colon without any trace of an ileocæcal valve, and the colon had a gradual curve throughout, there being no hepatic or splenic angle. The whole colon was provided with a mesentery. The appendix was present in the shape of a solid cord.

The Sigmoid Flexure opening into the Rectum on the Right Side.—This is a not uncommon congenital abnormality of the colon, and is probably present in about 4 per cent of all cases. Out of twenty-one newly-born infants dissected by Curling, the sigmoid joined the rectum on the right side in two. It is a condition well recognized by surgeons, as it is a cause of considerable embarrassment when attempting to perform a left inguinal colotomy in such cases.

Cæcum and Ascending Colon having a Mesentery.— Perhaps the commonest form of congenital abnormality of the colon is that in which the primitive arrangement of the peritoneum attaching the cæcum and ascending colon to the posterior abdominal wall has persisted. The condition varies from the cæcum alone having a short and complete mesentery, to that in which the cæcum and ascending colon, and half the transverse colon, have a common mesentery with the whole of the small intestine. Any condition between these two extremes may be met with, and that in which the cæcum has a short mesentery is comparatively common.

The cæcum in such cases may have a mesocolon five inches or more in length, and may be free to move about the abdominal cavity. In the cases in which it possesses, together with the ascending colon and right half of the transverse colon, a common mesentery with the small bowel, the cæcal angle of the colon (as it may be called) occupies a more or less central position in the abdomen.

This condition is very liable to result in the formation of a volvulus, often of a most complicated character. It will be further considered in the chapter on volvulus.

Treatment of Congenital Abnormalities.

Many of the congenital abnormalities of the colon which have been mentioned, such as complete atresia and absence of some portion of the large bowel, are quite incompatible with life, and are beyond the scope of surgical interference.

Most of the abnormalities are of practical interest chiefly because they give rise to difficulties in operating upon the colon, or because they are liable to result in volvulus. Apart from the complications which they may cause, they are seldom, if ever, diagnosed during life, and there is therefore no indication for attempting to correct them by surgical means.

The displacements of the cæcum and sigmoid are, however, of considerable practical importance to the surgeon, as should the necessity arise in such a case for the performance of a colotomy, their presence may render the operation most difficult, and sometimes impossible.

This was more especially the case in the days when lumbar colotomy was the usual operation, though considerable difficulty may result when performing an inguinal colotomy if the colon is not found in its usual position.

CONGENITAL DILATATION AND HYPERTROPHY OF THE COLON.

Probably the earliest recorded case, and certainly the first in which an operation was performed, is that reported by Dr. Bright in 1838. The real cause of the condition was detected by this astute observer, but he labelled the case "phantom tumour."

The condition is a very rare one, but probably not so uncommon as hospital records seem to prove. It is most frequently met with in children, but may be encountered at any age, as it is not necessarily fatal.

A great deal of uncertainty still exists as to the nature and causes of this disease, and it has been described under several names, such as "Hirschsprung's Disease," "Idiopathic Dilatation of the Colon," and "Congenital Dilatation of the Colon." The name used here, however, is that which best describes the condition.

Symptoms.

The chief symptoms are enormous distention of the abdomen, and severe and intractable constipation. In most of the cases one or both of these symptoms are noticed within a few days or weeks of birth.

In several instances no meconium has been passed for three or four days after birth, and there has subsequently been increasing difficulty in relieving the bowels.

Usually constipation is the first symptom, and distention of the abdomen is only manifest later; but in at least one instance the child was born with a distended abdomen, while in a case recorded by Walker and Griffiths, the distention was first noticed when the child was a few weeks old, and the constipation not till the age of three years.

The distention is the most marked characteristic. One child six months old measured 23½ inches in girth at the umbilicus; a boy aged eleven years had a girth of 3 feet 11 inches.

Formard has described a case in which the patient, a man, earned his living as a freak at shows. He was called the "balloon man" on account of the enormous size of his abdomen. In several cases, girls suffering from the disease have been suspected of pregnancy, owing to the size of their abdomens. The distention is mainly due to flatus, and the abdomen is always hyper-resonant. In extreme cases the splenic dullness is obliterated, and the liver dullness much diminished.

The distention is usually considerably diminished by an action of the bowels, but it is seldom completely relieved, and usually soon reappears.

When there is great distention, secondary symptoms occur from pressure upon other organs and upon the diaphragm. There may be marked shortness of breath and dyspnœa, the patient, during the height of the distention, being livid in the face from the embarrassed respiration. Palpitation may occur, from displacement of the heart, and the circulatory system may be seriously interfered with. The pressure results in great

HYPERTROPHY OF THE COLON

enlargement of the superficial veins of the abdomen, and in some cases has caused œdema of the legs. The kidneys may be damaged, and albuminuria is sometimes present.

The constipation is very intractable, the bowels often remaining unrelieved for days and weeks, in spite of the energetic employment of aperients and enemata.

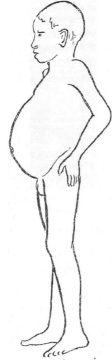

Fig. 24.—A boy, aged eleven, with congenital dilatation and hypertrophy of the colon.
(*After Osler.*)

In those cases which survive the first few years of life, there is a tendency for the symptoms to occur in periodic attacks, the patient often going months and even years without suffering any serious inconvenience from the condition; but constipation and unusual distention of the abdomen persist throughout. When an attack comes on, the patient becomes progressively more distended, and the bowels refuse to act. In some cases the patient goes weeks, and even months, without any action of the bowels. Sometimes the attack terminates in a copious action of the bowels which relieves the symptoms, to be followed in a few weeks or months by another similar attack.

The constipation may be so severe as to cause typical symptoms of intestinal obstruction ; the patient vomits, and suffers severe pain in the abdomen. Great coils of distended colon can be seen moving about through the stretched abdominal wall. In many cases an operation has been necessary to relieve the obstruction, and several patients have died from obstruction.

In a few cases the bowels have only been relieved by the administration of chloroform. One of the author's patients, a man of 23, was on three occasions relieved in this way, an immense mass of fæcal material coming away under the anæsthetic.

The constipation is usually characterized by long intervals during which there is no action of the bowels, followed by copious stools. Sometimes, however, there is spurious diarrhœa, small stools occurring at frequent intervals without any actual relief.

The health of the patient generally suffers considerably, and there is often serious emaciation and anæmia. The skin is discoloured, and there is marked toxæmia, often accompanied by a slight rise of temperature. In a few cases, however, except during the attacks of obstruction, the patient suffers no inconvenience, and even when the bowels have not acted for a long time there are no toxæmic symptoms.

Diagnosis.

This rests mainly upon the history of severe constipation accompanied by distention of the abdomen from birth or childhood, and the presence of an enormously dilated colon. Examination of the abdomen reveals great distention and tympanites. The lower angle of the ribs is flattened, and the chest pushed out at the sides, in extreme cases.

The abdominal veins are often enlarged. If the abdomen is examined while peristalsis is occurring in the colon, the huge coils of dilated bowel can often be seen moving, and may also be felt. In one case of the author's, the contractions of the dilated colon felt like those of the uterus in labour.

HYPERTROPHY OF THE COLON

Examination under the X rays, after a large enema containing bismuth, will often enable the dilated bowel to be seen. Most reliance, however, is to be placed on an examination with the sigmoidoscope, as the interior can then be observed. The interior of the colon under such circumstances looks like an immense sac almost filling the abdomen.

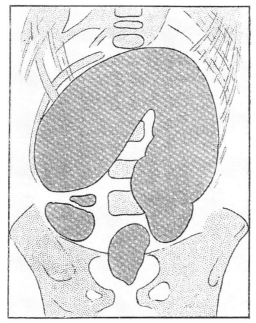

Fig. 25.—Skiagram in Dr. Carpenter's case of congenital dilatation of the colon after a large enema of Bismuth emulsion. It will be noticed that the ordinary shape of the colon has disappeared, and that there is one large U-shaped sac.

ETIOLOGY.

The condition is undoubtedly congenital in origin. This is clearly shown by the age tables, and by the fact that, even when the condition is present in an adult, there is almost without exception a history of the condition having begun in infancy or childhood. Several writers, who have drawn conclusions from a small number of cases, have been struck by an apparent age-gap in the cases, and have suggested that there exist two types of the condition, one occurring in children, which is congenital, and another, occurring in old people, which is acquired.

The following table, however, which is based upon a study of one hundred collected cases, disproves this :—

Ages.	Cases.
Under 5	24
5 to 10	16
10 to 20	14
20 to 30	11
30 to 40	7
40 to 50	8
50 to 60	5
60 to 70	6
Over 70	4
Not stated	5
Total	100

The greatest number of cases occur in infants, and the numbers steadily decrease up to old age. The condition is not necessarily fatal, and it seems certain that those occurring in the latter periods of life are congenital cases which have survived.

The condition is slightly commoner in males than in females, being in the proportion of three to two.

One would expect, if the condition were congenital, that associated congenital abnormalities would be common, but curiously enough this is apparently not so. Out of one hundred cases collected by the author, there were only fifteen in which there was any other congenital abnormality. In ten, there was a congenital abnormality of the anus, in two, a congenital stricture of the colon ; two were deaf mutes, and one an imbecile.

Several writers have attempted to prove that there is a connection between this condition and disease of the central nervous system, but there is no evidence of this. The cases of great dilatation of the colon which are often met with in the inmates of asylums are of an entirely different character, the bowel wall being thin and atrophied, whereas in this condition it is always hypertrophied. A further argument against the condition being due to a congenital neuro-muscular defect is, that powerful peristalsis undoubtedly occurs in the hypertrophied and dilated bowel. Nothnagel, recognizing that hypertrophy

HYPERTROPHY OF THE COLON

of the bowel wall is incompatible with a neuro-muscular defect, has suggested that there is such a defect of congenital origin in the lower part of the large bowel, and that the hypertrophy is a secondary effect occurring above it. There are, however, no pathological data to support this view.

The most probable explanation of this very puzzling condition seems to be, that there is some congenital abnormality which causes a partial or intermittent obstruction, and that the dilatation and hypertrophy are secondary to this. In support of this view we find that definite obstruction is present in some of the cases. Thus, out of the hundred cases already mentioned, obstruction was present in twenty-three.

CAUSES OF OBSTRUCTION.	CASES.
Congenital stricture of the rectum	11
Chronic volvulus of the sigmoid flexure	7
Angulation	2
Slight rectal narrowing	2
Congenital stricture of the sigmoid flexure	1
No obstruction found	77
TOTAL	100

Even when such a condition as a chronic volvulus exists, however, this may be a secondary consequence of the dilatation, and not its cause. The fact remains, that in the great majority of cases no obstruction of any kind is found, and also that in several the dilatation extended right down to the anus or to the middle of the rectum.

It seems possible that, owing to some abnormality of the mesentery of the sigmoid flexure, an angle or kink forms in this portion of the bowel which causes obstruction when the patient is in the erect position. An obstruction from this cause would, of course, not be obvious in the recumbent position, and would be undetectable at an operation or on the post-mortem table. There are, however, three cases on record in which the colon has again dilated after the dilated sigmoid had been resected, and a straight passage left between the end of the descending colon and the rectum. Such cases appear impossible of explanation at present. The most remarkable is that reported by Maurice Richardson.*

---

* *Boston Med. and Surg. Journ.*, Feb. 14, 1901.

Case.—The patient was a girl who had an enormous dilatation of the sigmoid flexure. The dilated sigmoid loop was resected, and the ends anastomosed so as to form a straight passage from the end of the descending colon to the rectum. A year and two months later the patient returned with fresh symptoms of obstruction and a distended abdomen, and on performing laparotomy it was found that a new coil of dilated bowel had formed, around the central portion of which the scar of the original anastomosis could be seen. Not only had the dilatation begun again here, but it had reached such dimensions that a new sigmoid flexure had formed which filled the pelvis and whole lower abdomen. This new dilated loop was again excised, but a year later the colon had again dilated at the same spot.

Morbid Anatomy.

The essential condition that is always present is great dilatation of the whole or part of the colon, accompanied by much thickening and hypertrophy of the dilated portion.

The dilatation is in all cases enormous, so that, as a rule, almost the entire abdominal cavity is occupied by the dilated portion of the colon, and on opening the abdomen nothing can be seen but the huge sac formed by the dilated bowel. The small intestines are not involved in the dilatation, but are usually found pushed into the back of the abdomen and collapsed.

The bowel is not only dilated, but also elongated, which results in its assuming abnormal and often acute flexures and kinks. This elongation is, however, limited to some extent by the mesentery, which prevents more than a certain limited amount of stretching in a longitudinal direction from taking place on that side of the bowel to which it is attached. The mesentery cannot, however, limit the longitudinal stretching of the colon on the side away from its attachment, and as a result this side becomes elongated to a much greater extent than the mesenteric side. The affected portion of colon becomes markedly convex in its longitudinal axis, and assumes a shape like that of the stomach, with a lesser and a greater curvature. Thus, the dilated portion of the colon is often spoken of as forming a huge pouch, or else as resembling the stomach.

A further result is that the mesentery becomes considerably shortened, as the peritoneum is separated by the dilatation of the colon between its layers. This shortening, combined with the deformity produced by elongation, causes the dilated bowel.

HYPERTROPHY OF THE COLON   69

to become much more fixed than is normally the case. The immobility of the colon is a well-marked feature when the abdomen is opened either at an operation for the relief of the condition, or post mortem. The dilated bowel cannot be pulled up or delivered out of the abdomen, or even moved about to any appreciable extent, unless it is first emptied of its contained gas. The dilated part of the colon varies in different cases. The entire colon, and the rectum to an inch above the anus, may be affected, or only one comparatively short portion.

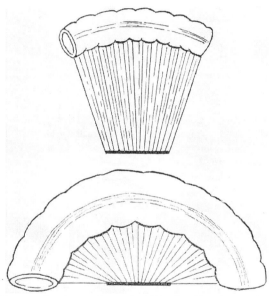

Fig. 26.—Diagram to show the secondary results of dilatation of the colon. As the colon becomes dilated, the mesocolon is shortened, and as the attachment of the mesocolon (shown by the black line) remains the same, the elongation of the colon which accompanies dilatation causes the curvature of the colon to be much exaggerated. The upper figure shows the normal, and the lower the dilated bowel.

In none of the cases I have collected have there been two separate and distinct dilatations in the same individual; and in none has the small bowel been affected.

The part most usually dilated is the sigmoid flexure alone: out of 100 cases, the dilatation involved the sigmoid alone in 51, while in 33 of the remainder it was involved together with other portions of the colon.

Thus, the sigmoid flexure was dilated in 84 out of 100 cases: the entire colon was dilated in 20, and in 9 of these the rectum was also involved in the dilatation; the transverse colon was the only part dilated in 2 cases, while it was involved with other parts in 36.

PARTS OF COLON AFFECTED.

Sigmoid ..	51
Whole colon	20
Hepatic flexure to rectum ..	11
Hepatic flexure to sigmoid ..	1
Splenic flexure to rectum ..	2
Cæcum to splenic flexure ..	4
Transverse colon ..	2
Descending colon	1

In some cases the dilatation begins and terminates abruptly; but in many, the transition from the dilated to the normal portion of the colon is funnel-shaped.

The dilatation of the bowel is rightly spoken of as enormous: in an infant thirteen months old the diameter of the dilated portion of the colon was 5 inches; and in a boy of ten the diameter was 6 inches.

In one of Dr. Hawkins's cases the circumference of the dilated portion of bowel was 43½ inches. In a case of the author's the diameter of the sigmoid flexure was estimated to be between 8 and 9 inches.

It is, of course, obvious that with such enormous dilatation and stretching of the bowel as occurs in these cases, the anatomical relationships of the affected portion of bowel are entirely altered, so that the apex of the sigmoid flexure may be found to lie under the liver. In some cases the thoracic organs have been considerably displaced, from the pushing up of the diaphragm and the widening of the angle of the lower ribs.

In addition to the dilatation, the bowel is also hypertrophied to a very marked degree, and this is quite as characteristic of the condition as the dilatation. The wall of the dilated portions of the colon is greatly thickened, in many cases being as much as a quarter of an inch in thickness, and so tough that it feels like thick leather.

The thickening extends to the peritoneum covering the bowel, but is chiefly found in the muscular coats. Both the longitudinal and circular fibres are hypertrophied, and on cutting

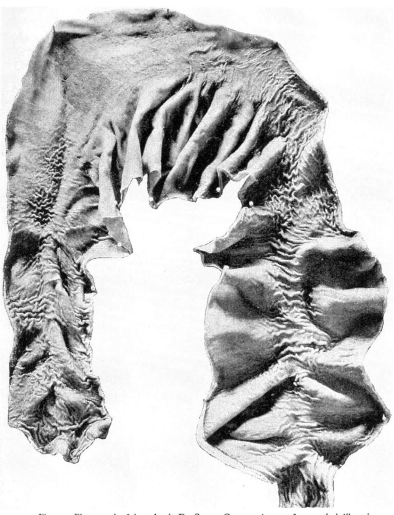

Fig. 27.—Photograph of the colon in Dr. George Carpenter's case of congenital dilatation in a child aged six months. [*Proc. Roy. Soc. Med.*, Dec., 1908, Vol. ii., No. 2, p. 39.]

HYPERTROPHY OF THE COLON

sections of the bowel-wall the muscle fibres can be seen to be increased both in size and in number.

The mucous membrane takes little if any part in the general hypertrophy, but there is some thickening of the submucosa.

This hypertrophy of the bowel-wall is not confined to the adult cases, but is also present in infants suffering from the condition.

In the specimen of Dr. Carpenter's case, illustrated in *Figs.* 27, 28, which was taken from an infant two months old, the wall of the dilated colon was an eighth of an inch thick, and felt like leather.

Contents of the Dilated Bowel. — These usually consist mainly of flatus, but very large quantities of fæcal material are present if the bowels have not acted for some time, and it is the accumulation of such material in large quantities which causes the ultimate acute symptoms in most cases. In

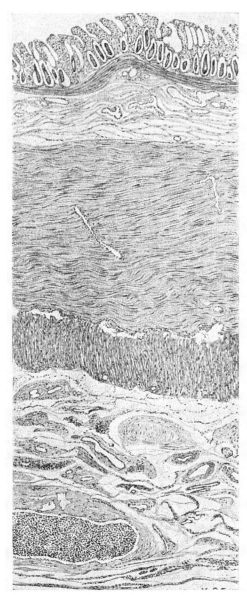

Fig. 28.—Microscopic section of the descending colon in the same case as *Fig.* 27.
[*Proc. Roy. Soc. Med.*, Dec., 1908, Vol. ii., No. 2, p. 39.]

several cases large fæcal calculi have been found in the dilated loop. In a case recorded by Tuppier there was a calculus weighing three pounds.

Secondary Changes in the Dilated Loop.—Stercoral ulceration in the dilated loop sometimes occurs, but is quite uncommon ; it was only present in twelve per cent of the author's cases. Death has resulted from perforation in a few of the cases.

Prognosis.

Out of the total cases, 63 died, and 32 are stated to have recovered ; the result is unknown in 5.

Of the cases said to have recovered, however, very few have been followed for more than a few months, so that the mortality is probably much higher than is represented by these figures.

Of the cases not operated upon there were 45, and of these 36 died and 9 recovered. Among the unoperated cases, therefore, the mortality is very high.

In the majority of cases death has occurred with symptoms of intestinal obstruction ; in some, from perforation and general peritonitis ; and in a few it was quite sudden, from no apparent cause. In one case death occurred while an enema was being administered, in two while the patient was in bed, and in one while the patient was getting out of bed. In a good many cases it has apparently resulted from some operation undertaken for the relief of the condition.

Several of the patients have died from acute obstruction due to a volvulus of the dilated coil.

Toxæmia and exhaustion, or marasmus, have been the cause of death in some cases, especially in children and infants.

It is a mistake, however, to suppose that the condition is necessarily fatal if left alone, for in quite a number of instances children suffering from the condition have grown up and reached adult age.

In the author's collected cases, there were ten who had lived to over 60 years of age. Usually, however, the condition proves fatal in the first few years of life.

Treatment of Congenital Dilatation and Hypertrophy of the Colon.

Non-operative Treatment.—The non-operative treatment of this condition consists principally in getting the bowels to act

HYPERTROPHY OF THE COLON

regularly by the administration of enemas and aperients. Aperients are usually of little use, and enemata will have to be employed. Large enemata, if carefully administered, will, in some cases, keep the patient in comparative comfort; but they will have to be used daily in order to prevent accumulation of fæces in the dilated bowel. Large doses of magnesium sulphate will sometimes relieve the constipation by rendering the contents of the colon fluid. Intestinal muscle stimulants such as strychnine, nux vomica, and ergot may be tried, and abdominal massage and application of the galvanic current will often allay the symptoms for a time.

When these measures fail, recourse must be had to operation, which in most cases becomes necessary sooner or later.

OPERATIVE TREATMENT.—Whenever possible, operation should be avoided when there are obstructive symptoms and the dilated bowel is loaded with solid fæces. Every effort should first be made to empty the bowel: even then the dilated colon is not easy to deal with, and when loaded with many pounds of semi-solid fæces the greatest difficulty may be experienced.

Colotomy.—The record of cases operated upon show that the mortality attending colotomy for this condition is very high, higher in fact than for any other procedure. Thus, out of fourteen cases treated by colotomy, eleven died. This might to some extent be accounted for if the colotomy was done only for the relief of obstruction where acute symptoms were present; but the cases show that, even when colotomy was done where no acute symptoms existed at the time of operation, it often proved fatal. Death occurred in most cases from general peritonitis following the operation, and it was found at the post-mortem examination that the bowel had torn away from the abdominal wall, or leaked. The reason for this is obvious: an artificial anus made into a huge pouch of bowel, such as is usually present in these cases, is a very different thing from an ordinary colotomy operation performed on normal bowel. The dilated loop is large and heavy, and a very serious drag occurs upon the sutures uniting it to the abdominal wall. The result is that the colon usually tears away, and causes general peritonitis from leakage into the peritoneal cavity.

The formation of a spur is, of course, impossible, and if colotomy has to be done, it should be by the lumbar route.

Quite apart from the fatal results which have followed

colotomy in these cases, this operation frequently fails to relieve the obstruction. In quite a number of cases the bowels would not act through the colotomy opening, and the author has only been able to find two in which any benefit was obtained from the operation.

We must conclude that colotomy is both a dangerous and unsatisfactory operation in these cases, and should not be performed except for the relief of urgent obstruction, when the bowel above the dilated portion should be opened or lumbar colotomy performed.

Resection of the Dilated Portion of the Colon.—This is the operation which has been attended with the best results in these cases, and in spite of the difficulty of resecting such enormously dilated bowel, it has not been attended by a high mortality.

In all but two of the collected cases in which this operation was performed, the dilatation was confined to the pelvic colon. In one case, however, the entire colon was successfully resected for this condition.

In most of the cases where resection has been successfully performed, the patient has completely recovered; but in at least three instances the dilatation has recurred after resection. In Dr. Richardson's case, a second resection of the dilated colon was done, but the condition again recurred. Even resection of the dilated bowel cannot, therefore, be depended upon to cure the condition, as some remaining portion of the bowel may again dilate, and cause the same symptoms as before. In those cases, however, where the condition recurred, the portion in which the re-dilatation took place included the line of anastomosis, and this rather suggests that possibly if the colon had in the first instance been more widely resected, there would have been no recurrence.

When the dilatation is confined to the sigmoid flexure, resection of the dilated loop, going as wide as possible of the affected portion, seems to be the best method of treatment.

When the whole or the greater portion of the colon is involved, the operation must be attended by such difficulties, owing to the size and fixity of the bowel, that it is doubtful if it is justifiable, and a preliminary short-circuiting operation is preferable.

In one case I performed appendicostomy for this condition. The operation was done in the hope of being able to prevent accumulation in the enormously distended sigmoid by washing out the whole colon daily with water through the appendix. The patient, a man of 22, was quite well between the attacks of obstruction from which he suffered, and it did not seem justifiable to subject him to the danger of excision of the enormous loop of dilated bowel, unless every other method failed.

After the operation it was found possible for him to keep his dilated sigmoid practically empty by daily washing it through from the appendix.

A year after operation he was still well. He washed out the colon daily through the appendicostomy opening, and, although during that time there had twice been considerable difficulty in getting the bowels open, the threatened obstruction had, on both occasions, been overcome by the injection of warm water into the cæcum.

It would seem as if the operation were well worth a trial before proceeding to more serious measures.

Ileo-sigmoidostomy has been performed in a few cases; but, although it may afford temporary relief, it cannot cure the condition unless followed by resection of the dilated loop. The operation of narrowing the dilated bowel by means of Lembert sutures, in a similar manner to the operation of gastroplication for the relief of gastric dilatation, has also been tried, but no good results have followed it. Fixation of the colon has been similarly unsuccessful.

REFERENCES.

KEITH.—*Lond. Hosp. Museum Cat.* Nos. 1238, 1238a, c, d, and 1239.
TREVES.—*Intestinal Obst.* 1899, 232.
LOCKWOOD.—*Brit. Med. Jour.* 1882, ii. 574, and *Barts. Hosp. Reps.* Vol. 19.
ROLLESTON.—*Path. Trans.* 1891, 122.
FITZ.—*Amer. Jour. Med. Sci.* Aug., 1889.
TREVES.—*Lancet*, 1898, i. 276.
OSLER.—*Johns Hopkins Hosp. Bull.* iv. 30.
GOODHART.—*Clin. Trans.* 1880, xiv. 84.
ROLLESTON and HAYWARD.—*Trans. Clin. Soc.* 1896, xxix. 201.
FORMARD.—*Annals of the Universal Med. Sci.* Vol. i. 93.
HIRSCHSPRUNG.—*Annals of the Universal Med. Sci.* Vol. i. 1893.
JACOBY.—*Archiv. Pediatrics*, 1893, Vol. x. 440.
WOOLMER.—*Brit. Med. Jour.* 1889, 1330.

Chapter VII.

VOLVULUS OF THE COLON.

By a volvulus we understand a condition in which some portion of the colon has twisted upon itself or around its mesentery. There are several kinds of volvulus, depending upon the part of the colon involved, and the nature and direction of the twist. It is obvious that volvulus can only occur where the colon has a mesentery, and the only part of the colon which normally possesses a mesentery sufficiently long to allow the colon to twist is the pelvic colon; but abnormally, other portions of the colon may have a long mesentery, and then may become twisted. Volvulus forms about 4 per cent of all cases of intestinal obstruction.

From a clinical standpoint we may divide the cases of volvulus into *acute volvulus*, in which the twist forms suddenly and causes complete obstruction and strangulation of the involved gut; and *chronic volvulus*, in which the twist is not complete and does not cause strangulation, though it produces temporary obstruction.

Symptoms.

Acute Volvulus.—This is the commoner condition, and the symptoms are those of acute intestinal obstruction. They usually commence quite suddenly, with abdominal pain and colic. The pain is often severe, and when first seen the patient is frequently doubled up in bed and groaning with the pain, which comes on in spasms. There is usually absolute constipation, but exceptionally there may be straining and tenesmus, with the passage of small liquid stools and mucus. Vomiting is not a marked feature of obstruction from this cause, and not infrequently is absent altogether. The most marked feature of the symptoms is distention of the abdomen. This occurs rapidly, and soon reaches great dimensions. The abdomen is tense, the diaphragm pushed up, and the respiration may be much embarrassed. The abdomen is

VOLVULUS OF THE COLON

hyper-resonant. The distention usually is so great that but little can be made out in the abdomen, and it is not possible to locate the trouble to any particular area.

Another characteristic symptom is early and acute tenderness of the abdomen. Collapse, with paleness of the skin and a feeble pulse, occurs after the condition has existed for some time, but it does not appear so early, nor is it so well marked as in many other forms of intra-abdominal trouble.

In those cases where the cæcum is involved in the volvulus, the onset of the symptoms is usually somewhat slower, and vomiting is almost invariably present.

As a rule the pain in volvulus is more or less correctly localized to the area overlying the lesion, and this may be used as a guide in diagnosis. Acute and severe toxæmia is usually present in acute volvulus, and in the later stages the patient presents all the symptoms of acute poisoning from the contents of his own intestine. The progress of the case varies considerably. Occasionally it is very rapid; thus Mr. Heath recently reported a case in which a volvulus of the sigmoid became completely gangrenous in thirty hours, and even more rapid cases of gangrene than this have occurred. On the other hand, the symptoms of volvulus may exist for several days, and yet at the operation the volvulus is not found to be gangrenous; the condition, of course, depends on the severity and tightness of the twist.

In volvulus of the ileocæcal angle the symptoms may be very acute and death occur early, owing to the large mass of bowel which is strangulated. Thus in a case described by Mr. Burgess,[*] death occurred in sixteen hours from the onset of symptoms. The patient was a boy aged 8, in whom the volvulus included the whole of the intestine, from the duodenum to the middle of the ascending colon.

CHRONIC VOLVULUS. — There are usually recurring attacks of obstruction, with pain and constipation. In a typical case the patient has repeated attacks of obstruction at varying intervals, which either pass off after a short time, or are relieved by the administration of an enema. During the attacks the symptoms are often alarming, the abdomen is distended, the bowels will not act, and there is great pain in the abdomen. The attack, however, passes off, only to recur at

---

[*] *Lancet*, Dec., 1902.

some later period. In other cases there are no symptoms of acute obstruction at any time, but the patient has attacks of obstinate constipation lasting for several days, when the bowels refuse to act and there is abdominal discomfort. Between the attacks he may be quite well, though occasionally there is a complaint of dull pain in the back or in the abdomen. These cases not infrequently culminate in acute and fatal obstruction.

In chronic volvulus of the cæcal angle, frequent and recurring attacks of slight obstruction, with vomiting and distention, are not uncommon, and in some cases attacks have continued for several years before an acute and serious crisis necessitating operation has occurred. In some cases of chronic or recurring volvulus, the symptoms are very obscure, and it is only as the result of an exploratory operation that the true nature of the condition is made clear. It is probable that in many of these the twist only occurs while the patient is in the erect position. Thus patients suffering from this condition sometimes state that they can only pass flatus when lying down, and the author once operated upon a patient who said he was only able to pass flatus by going on his hands and knees. There is often great difficulty in getting the bowels to act, and aperients are frequently useless. Enemas, by distending the bowel and so partly untwisting it, often give relief when aperients will not do so. Many patients with chronic volvulus complain of a dragging pain in the back when standing or walking, and of vague abdominal discomfort. Their symptoms are often indefinite and vague, and as a result are often quite unnecessarily put down to neurasthenia.

The diagnosis is often difficult as regards the cause of the obstruction; but volvulus may be suspected when in a case of acute intestinal obstruction we find marked distention and no vomiting. The patients are often elderly, and the condition is very rare in children and young adults. It also appears to be more common in men than in women.

The cases in which the cæcal angle is involved may cause great difficulty in diagnosis; and even when the abdomen is opened, the complicated arrangement of the parts may render it almost impossible to ascertain what has occurred.

Etiology.

Predisposing Causes.—1. Mal-development of the peritoneum attaching the bowel to the posterior abdominal wall, or of the

THE COLON

mesentery. This is the usual predisposing cause of compound and cæcal volvuli.

2. Alteration in the normal proportions between the length of the mesentery and of its base of attachment. Thus the mesentery may be too long, so that it readily twists about its base of attachment as an axis. The elongation of the mesentery may be congenital or acquired. Or the base of attachment may be too short, which produces a similar condition, and allows the loop to twist around its base. This is a common cause of sigmoid volvulus, the shortening of the base of attachment being due to chronic inflammation of the mesentery.

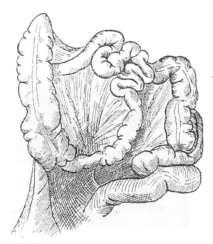

Fig. 29.—A specimen showing a common mesentery to the cæcum and ileum. This is a congenital abnormality which predisposes to volvulus of the cæcal angle. The cæcum has been turned up. (*After Alglave.*)

3. Adhesions or contractions in the mesentery which draw it into a pedicle and allow the distal portion of the loop to twist around the narrowed portion.

4. Adhesions of part of the colon to some other portion of the intestine or to another viscus or structure. This may result in some other part of the colon becoming twisted round the adherent portion as an axis.

The predisposing causes of volvulus may exist for years without causing obstruction, and some further or exciting cause is necessary before serious symptoms occur.

The exciting causes of volvulus are not well known, and are often not evident. Loading of the bowel with fæces, and distention with flatus, may act as exciting causes by forcing the bowel to assume a fresh position in the abdominal cavity. Sudden strain, and external violence, often appear to act as exciting causes.

The best examples of volvulus due to congenital abnormalities of the mesentery occur at the ileocæcal angle.

Elongation of the mesentery is a not uncommon cause of volvulus of the sigmoid. In some instances the mesosigmoid is

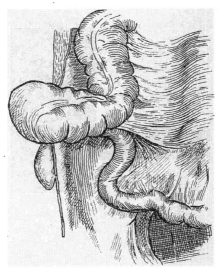

Fig. 30.—A congenital abnormality of the peritoneum. The cæcum is freely movable, and the last few inches of the ileum are fixed. This may result in volvulus. *(After Alglave.)*

congenitally too long. More usually the elongation has resulted from overloading of the sigmoid from constipation of long standing, and consequent stretching of the mesosigmoid from the weight of the loaded loop.

In a case recorded by Bonuzzi, the mesosigmoid was four times its normal length, and in one of my own cases it was more than twice its normal length. In Bonuzzi's case, complete volvulus had resulted, while in mine a partial volvulus occurred and caused intermittent obstruction. I have been able to find one case of volvulus of the sigmoid in a child two years and four months old. It seems probable that in this patient, and the two mentioned above, the elongation of the mesosigmoid was congenital. In volvulus of the cæcal angle, the abnormality of the mesentery is always congenital.

Shortening of the base of attachment of the mesentery has been described as congenital; but there is no proof of this, and it seems more probable that it is always acquired. The usual condition is one of cicatricial contraction of the peritoneum from chronic inflammation in the mesosigmoid. Such chronic inflammation is a not uncommon result of constipation. Bands of thickening in the peritoneum can often be demonstrated, or actual adhesions involving the base of the mesosigmoid can be seen.

Tumours in the mesentery may also cause shortening, and cases are recorded of volvulus occurring as the result of a lipoma or sarcoma in the mesentery. Glands which have caseated and subsequently caused a cicatrix are also met with as a cause of volvulus.

General Pathology.

Volvulus of the colon is most common in the sigmoid flexure. Thus out of seventeen cases at the London Hospital, twelve were of the sigmoid flexure, and five of the cæcum. Other figures agree closely with this. After the sigmoid flexure the commonest situation for volvulus of the colon is the cæcum or ileocæcal angle, and this can only occur as the result of a congenital abnormality of the peritoneum. The same applies to volvulus of any other portion of the colon; but such conditions are very rare. I have found one case of volvulus of the splenic angle which was operated upon by Mr. Littlewood. The volvulus consisted of the splenic flexure, part of the transverse colon, the descending colon, and part of the sigmoid flexure. This portion of the colon had a mesentery five inches long. The entire splenic angle had twisted upon itself and caused obstruction of the middle of the transverse colon. Such cases must be very rare, as I have been unable to find another instance. A volvulus of the descending colon is reported by Crisp. The transverse colon is not uncommonly involved in cases of compound and cæcal volvulus, but it cannot become twisted on itself.

The varieties are very numerous, and the most curious

and varied pathological conditions are found. Two distinct pathological types of volvulus or twisting occur :—

(*a*). When the twist has occluded the vessels in the pedicle of the loop : that is, when the blood-supply to the affected bowel is arrested.

(*b*). When the blood-supply of the affected loop is still adequate, but the bowel lumen is partly or entirely obstructed.

The affected loop of bowel (in condition *a*) becomes dark in colour, the walls become œdematous, and serum and, later, blood, is exuded from the vessels into the lumen of the bowel, and also into the peritoneal cavity. This exudation of blood-stained serum is due to rupture of the finer capillaries and to intense inflammation. The affected loop also becomes greatly distended with gas, and this is one of the most marked features of volvulus. The distention occurs very rapidly, and reaches great proportions. The gas causing the distention is chiefly carbon dioxide, and arises from the fermentation of the fæcal contents of the bowel. This gas is normally formed in the bowel, but is absorbed and carried away by the blood-stream, and also passed on by peristalsis, almost as fast as it forms. When the blood-stream is arrested, and the bowel lumen is at the same time closed, the gas accumulates in the twisted loop, and causes the distention.

In the experiments which I performed upon cats (*page* 33) it was found that distention did not occur unless the venous blood-stream was arrested. If a loop of the colon was thoroughly cleaned out with water before it was twisted, or before the blood-supply was arrested by ligature, distention did not occur, though the phenomena of strangulation did. This proves that the formation of gas is not due to the strangulation, but is simply the result of fermentation of the fæcal contents, and that the distention results from unrestrained fermentation in the affected loop, the gas so formed not being absorbed by the blood or being able to pass into other parts of the bowel. The pathological changes which occur in complete volvulus (condition *a*) differ in no important respect from ordinary strangulation, such as occurs in strangulated hernia. The probable reason that distention is more marked in the case of volvulus is that fermentation more readily occurs in the colon. The conditions for bacterial action in the colon are aerobic, while in the greater part of the small intestine they are anaerobic. Gangrene of the bowel

THE COLON

ultimately occurs, and general peritonitis may be the cause of death.

In partial volvulus (condition *b*), the pathological conditions are the same as in other forms of obstruction of the colon where strangulation is not present. Distention is not a marked feature.

Violent peristalsis occurs above the twist, and a certain amount of distention with fæces and gas in the bowel above. If the partial volvulus is intermittent and lasts for a long time, hypertrophy of the bowel above will take place, as in the case of any other form of partial obstruction.

Volvulus of the Pelvic Colon.—This is the commonest form of volvulus. The predisposing cause in most cases is elongation of the pelvic mesocolon from chronic overloading of this portion of the bowel, as commonly occurs in constipation. Meso-sigmoiditis, with contraction and narrowing of the mesentery, is a not uncommon contributory cause. The twist may occur in either direction, but the commonest is the clockwise direction with the rectum behind the upper limb of the loop. The distention of the twisted loop rapidly becomes extreme, and the sigmoid may fill the entire abdominal cavity, and even displace the thoracic organs.

Rupture of the loop rarely occurs, but hæmorrhages into it are common, and after a day or two micro-organisms apparently pass through the bowel wall of the volvulus and cause septic infection of the peritoneum. Volvulus of the sigmoid flexure sometimes occurs in association with congenital dilatation of the colon, but this has already been referred to.

Volvulus of the pelvic colon is usually considered a condition of late life; but I have met with one case in a child aged two years and four months.

Volvulus of the Cæcum and Ascending Colon (cæcal angle).—Several varieties of this form of volvulus have been described, but the only difference is in the length of the loop. It can only occur if the cæcum possesses a mesentery, and the parts involved in the volvulus will depend upon the length and attachments of this mesentery.

Several drawings are given of abnormal arrangements of the peritoneum covering the cæcum and ascending colon (*Figs.* 29 and 30), and it will be seen that any condition may occur between that of a cæcum having a short mesentery, and one in which the cæcum, ascending colon, and part of the transverse colon have a common mesentery with the whole of the small bowel. In the former case the cæcum alone may become twisted upon the termination of the ileum and the commencement of the ascending colon; in the latter, the cæcum, ascending colon, and ileum may become twisted around the transverse colon and jejunum or duodenum. There are examples of both these conditions.

Usually the twist occurs around the ileum as an axis, the heavier and larger portion of the bowel twisting round the smaller and lighter. In Dr. Whipham's case, the entire small bowel, together with the cæcum and ascending colon, had twisted round the jejunum. In another case the cæcum, ascending colon, and transverse colon had twisted round the ileum.

The twist may occur in either direction, but the commonest condition seems to be from left to right. By this I mean in the anti-clockwise direction, the cæcum passing behind the mesentery and from the right to the left side of the abdomen.

In speaking of the development of the colon, I mentioned that, in the earliest stages, the whole alimentary canal possessed only one straight mesentery or peritoneal attachment to the posterior abdominal wall. This primitive condition is found in the three-months fœtus, and also in some of the lower primates (notably *Lemur coronatus*). At first, this single mesentery lies vertically in the median line, and the alimentary canal is a single straight tube from one end of the body to the other. Very rapidly, however, the alimentary canal lengthens, and in so doing becomes thrown into folds. At the same time new peritoneal connections or attachments are formed between these folds and the posterior abdominal wall.

The cæcum passes across to the right flank, and later, downwards into the right iliac fossa; at the same time it loses its original mesentery and becomes fixed in the right iliac fossa in the condition normally found in man. There do not appear to be any cases in which the early primitive condition has persisted in its entirety,—that is to say, where the whole colon shares a common mesentery with the small bowel. But, rarely, the cæcum, ascending, and part of the transverse colon, are found to have a common mesentery with the whole of the small bowel up to the duodenum.

It is quite obvious that when this arrangement of the mesentery persists as a congenital abnormality, there is always a possibility

THE COLON

of the large mass of bowel which is suspended from a single and comparatively narrow mesenteric attachment becoming twisted around its axis and causing a volvulus. That it does not always so result is shown by the fact that this condition of the mesentery is sometimes found post mortem in elderly patients dying from other diseases.

The pathological condition presented in these cases of volvulus

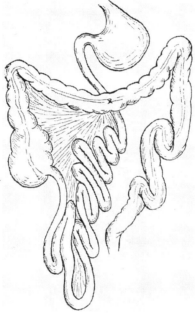

Fig. 31.—Diagram showing the condition present when there is a common mesentery to the ileum and the right side of the colon. Volvulus is liable to occur, the twist taking place round the point marked X.

of the cæcal angle is often most complex. As a rule an operation is performed for the relief of intestinal obstruction, and on opening the abdomen the cæcum is found not to be in its normal position. The position varies considerably; most commonly it is found somewhere on the left side of the abdomen, either below the stomach or over the left kidney : it will depend upon the length of the adventitious cæcal mesentery and upon the extent of the twist.

The most noticeable thing on examining the abdominal cavity is the complete emptiness of the right iliac fossa, and it is this which, as a rule, first draws attention to the nature of the condition. The axis of the twist is usually the small bowel; but the part concerned depends upon the degree of abnormality of the peritoneum present. Thus the ileum may form the axis of rotation, or it may be the jejunum, and in two cases the duodenum formed the axis of the volvulus.

Where the complete condition exists, the twist occurs around the base of attachment of the common mesentery, the duodenum, and the centre of the transverse colon : the actual axis is usually the superior mesenteric artery, which here passes forward between the layers of the mesentery, and which supplies practically the whole area of bowel forming the volvulus. In most cases the rotation is in an anti-clockwise direction (as looked at from below), i.e., the ileum passes forward and to the right, while the cæcum passes backwards and to the left. The twist very rarely occurs in the opposite direction. A reference to the diagram will at once show why the rotation is usually in the former direction. When the parts are lying in their normal position and no volvulus has occurred, it will be seen that a half-twist in the anti-clockwise direction already exists; so that an accidental half-twist in that direction will cause a volvulus of the entire loop, while a similar half-twist in the opposite direction will simply undo the normal half-twist.

In order, therefore, for this condition to occur from a twist in the clockwise direction, the loop of bowel would have to twist through a circle and a half, while to produce a volvulus in the opposite direction it will have to rotate through half a circle only. The probabilities, therefore, are much greater of a volvulus being produced in one direction than in the other.

In only two of the twenty-nine cases I have collected was the twist in a clockwise direction. In eighteen of the twenty-nine cases there was a common mesentery to the whole of the ileum, cæcum, ascending colon, and part of the transverse colon. In seven cases the cæcum had a mesentery, and was free to move about. In three the cæcum and ascending colon had a long mesentery.

In one case there was a compound volvulus resulting in a most complicated condition. The sigmoid flexure was twisted round the ileum, cæcum, and ascending colon from left to right. One

THE COLON

would suppose that this form of volvulus, owing to its congenital origin, would occur most frequently in children and infants, but this is apparently not so. Most of the cases are in adults, and the condition is most frequent between the ages of twenty and forty.

The following table shows the age incidence in twenty-seven cases. There were three cases in infants, the youngest being four days old, while the oldest patient was seventy-two :—

	Cases.
Under 5 years of age	3
Between 5 and 20	6
Between 20 and 40	10
Between 40 and 60	5
Over 60	3

The average age was 31.

If there is a common mesentery to the ascending colon, cæcum, and small bowel, the condition of the patient when volvulus occurs is a very serious one, owing to the great length of the bowel involved in the twist.

Compound Volvulus.—Many of the cases of cæcal volvulus in which the ileum, cæcum, and ascending colon were involved, have been described as compound. But if the term is to be retained, it should be reserved for cases in which either two separate and distinct twists have taken place in different portions of the bowel, as, for instance, where there is a volvulus in the small bowel and another in the sigmoid, or where a portion of the small intestine has become twisted round the sigmoid flexure, or vice versa. Karl Richter has recorded three cases in which there was a volvulus of the small intestine and another of the sigmoid flexure. The small intestine may become twisted round the sigmoid flexure, but more commonly the former acts as the axis and the sigmoid is twisted round it.

Leichenstein collected twenty-one cases of this form of compound volvulus. In twelve of these the loop of small intestine formed the axis, and the sigmoid was twisted round it from left to right, and from before backwards. In the remaining cases the sigmoid was twisted round the small intestine in the opposite direction.

TREATMENT.

In cases of acute or complete volvulus, immediate operation affords the only hope of saving the patient's life, and much of the success of the operation depends upon its being performed as soon as possible after the occurrence of the twist. Volvulus cannot always be diagnosed apart from operation, but we can always diagnose the presence of acute obstruction, and this is sufficient indication for immediate operation.

The abdomen must be opened, and the distended loop pulled out. Although it is excellent practice when operating upon the abdominal viscera not to expose the gut more than is absolutely necessary—and this is particularly advisable in acute cases—at the same time, directly a volvulus has been detected it is useless to attempt to deal with it inside the abdominal cavity through a small incision. A free opening should be made and the entire involved loop pulled out. This is more especially necessary in dealing with volvulus of the cæcal angle, or compound volvulus, for these are so complicated that, if a big incision is not made and the whole mass brought out, it is more than probable the reduction of the twist will be incomplete.

The distended loop or loops, having been delivered, must next be unravelled, and the colon carefully examined to make certain that the obstruction has been completely removed. If the volvulus has only existed a few hours, it will probably be safe to return it and close the abdomen. If, however, there is much distention, or if it has existed for more than a few hours, the coil must be emptied of its contents, and drained by establishing an artificial anus. This is rendered necessary by the fact that the twisted coil almost certainly contains highly virulent pathogenic organisms and toxins, and its walls are allowing these to pass into the circulation, and also into the peritoneal cavity. The bowel is, moreover, at any rate temporarily, paralyzed : if it is simply untwisted and returned, many of the patients will die within the next forty-eight hours from intense toxæmia or peritonitis. If possible the distended loop should be washed out, and a Paul's tube tied into it to allow of the contents draining freely away.

Nothing more can be done at the first operation ; but if the patient recovers, the advisability of performing another operation to prevent recurrence should be considered, because the predisposing cause of the volvulus is still present, and a recurrence is very probable if nothing further is attempted.

It is difficult to trace cases of volvulus in order to ascertain if recurrence has occurred in those cases where the bowel has

THE COLON

simply been untwisted; most writers, however, agree that it is common, and I have been able to find several cases in which the after-history showed recurrence to have taken place.

One patient, a man aged 21, had a volvulus of the sigmoid. This was untwisted and colotomy performed. He recovered, and the colotomy opening closed. Two years later, he again got a volvulus of the sigmoid flexure: on this occasion the sigmoid was resected, and he remained well.

In another case, that of a man aged 63, with volvulus of the sigmoid, the volvulus was untwisted and the colon fixed by forming an artificial anus. The patient recovered, and the opening was allowed to close. A year later the volvulus recurred, and at the operation the adhesions were found to have entirely disappeared. The sigmoid was again untwisted. Eleven months later he had for the third time to be operated upon for a volvulus of the sigmoid.

METHODS OF PREVENTING RECURRENCE.—Various operations have been advised in order to prevent a recurrence of the volvulus. Braun suggested stitching the loop to the abdominal wall, or in the case of the sigmoid, to the iliac fossa.

Senn in two cases shortened the mesentery by folding it upon itself in a direction parallel to the bowel, and sutured the apex of the loop to the root of the mesentery. He stated that no recurrence occurred in either of these cases. One would suppose that the formation of an artificial anus, and the adhesions resulting from this procedure, would be an efficient preventive of recurrence of the volvulus; but this is not so, as the cases just quoted prove.

Similarly, fixation of the loop by sutures to the abdominal wall or iliac fossa, as suggested by Braun, is useless; it could hardly be as effective as the formation of an artificial anus, and, moreover, in three cases where this was done, recurrence occurred a year later.

Shortening of the mesosigmoid offers a better prospect, but the best method of preventing recurrence, and probably the only certain one, is excision of the sigmoid loop. This may be done at the time of the first operation if Paul's method is adopted of resecting the bowel and tying a Paul's tube into either end. If this is not considered advisable at the time of the first operation, a second should be done after the patient has recovered from the obstruction, and the loop excised. The ends may either be united end to end, or brought out and the spur divided later with an enterotome.

TREATMENT WHEN THE COLON IS GANGRENOUS.—If the volvulus is found to be gangrenous, excision is the only remedy, and the best chance of recovery will be secured by tying a Paul's tube into each end of the colon after resection, and bringing the ends out.

TREATMENT OF VOLVULUS OF THE CÆCAL ANGLE.—This operation is much more difficult than in the case of the sigmoid, owing partly to the fact that, as a result of the obstruction being higher up and involving a large amount of bowel, the patient is probably more acutely ill, but chiefly to the very complicated condition of affairs that is found on opening the abdomen, and the difficulty of ascertaining exactly what has happened.

The greatest difficulty may be experienced in untwisting the bowel, and the operation necessarily takes some time.

Of the twenty-nine cases collected by the author, seventeen were operated upon. In two, nothing was done beyond opening the abdomen and closing it again; both died. The following table shows what was done, and the result, in the remaining fifteen cases:—

	CASES.	DIED.	RECOVERED.
Untwisting of volvulus	9	5	4
Enterostomy	5	5	—
Excision	1	—	1
TOTAL	15	10	5

It will be seen that out of the total seventeen cases, only five recovered. In two of the cases in which the volvulus was untwisted, it was found post mortem that reduction had been incomplete. Enterostomy is evidently useless, as all the cases so treated died, and it is necessary to untwist or excise the volvulus if the patient is to have any chance of recovery.

Excision is a formidable operation in such cases as these, as the patient is dangerously ill already, and a considerable length of bowel will have to be removed. In some cases it would be impossible, since it would involve removal of the greater part or even the whole of the small bowel.

A case has been recorded in which the twisted loop was gangrenous and 80 cms. of bowel were resected, the patient

THE COLON

recovering. This case is a remarkable one, and shows that excision is justifiable, even when dealing with such a severe lesion as a gangrenous volvulus of the cæcal angle of the colon.

TREATMENT OF CHRONIC VOLVULUS.—This condition does not call for treatment because there is acute obstruction, and it can seldom be diagnosed with certainty without opening the abdomen. It is very unlikely that a volvulus will be found at the operation ; but a careful examination will reveal an abnormal condition of the mesocolon allowing a partial or complete twist of the colon to take place.

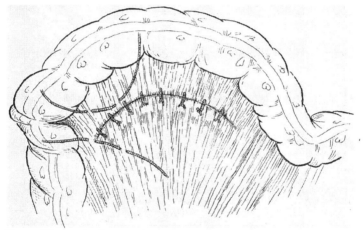

Fig. 32.—Diagram showing method of shortening the mesocolon by Lembert sutures. The stitches pass through the outer peritoneum only, so as not to constrict the vessels. The method of passing additional sutures in order to remove a kink is also shown.

The most effectual means of dealing with the condition is to get rid of the loop of colon by excision and end-to-end anastomosis. This is, however, a somewhat serious operation, and a good result may often be obtained by measures involving less risk. Since the condition is in most cases due to a deformity of the mesentery, the indication is to correct this, and the procedure which has most to recommend it is to shorten the mesocolon by means of suitably placed sutures.

Another method which is sometimes used is to anchor the apex of the loop to the parietal peritoneum by means of sutures ; but while this may succeed in the case of the cæcal angle, it is more than likely to fail when the sigmoid flexure is involved, owing to the weight of this part of the colon when filled with solid fæces causing the adhesions to tear away.

OPERATION FOR SHORTENING THE MESOCOLON.—The loop of bowel forming the volvulus is drawn out of the abdominal wound, and held towards the inner side of the wound by an assistant, so as to put the mesocolon slightly on the stretch. A row of Lembert sutures are then inserted, taking up the peritoneum only, right across the mesocolon to within a short distance of the bowel on each side. These sutures should be inserted on the outer or iliac side of the mesocolon, and when inserting them, care should be taken to avoid injuring any blood-vessels. When this row of sutures is tied, it should form a pleat in the mesocolon. A second similar row of sutures is then inserted over the first, so as to shorten still further the mesentery, and if necessary a third row. After the sutures have been inserted it will be found that a kink has been formed in the colon at either end of the suture line. To get rid of this a few more Lembert sutures should be inserted parallel to the bowel wall and opposite any such kink (see *Fig.* 32). If the sutures are properly placed the kink can be straightened out. It is, of course, necessary to see that the blood-supply of the loop has not been interfered with by the suturing, but if the stitches have been carefully placed there should be no difficulty.

In one patient on whom I performed this operation, the mesocolon was over eight inches long, and was reduced to three and a half inches by the suturing. Previous to operation he had suffered severely from constipation, and could only relieve his bowels by means of large enemata. Afterwards the bowels acted normally, and the result was excellent.

REFERENCES.

HUTCHINSON.—*Clin. Jour.* June 5, 1907.
TUTTLE.—*New York Med. Jour.* Mar. 14, 1908.
DELATOUR.—*Annals of Surg.* Nov. 1905.
HANDFIELD-JONES.—*Med. Times and Gaz.* Jan. 6, 1872.
FAGGE.—*Guy's Hosp. Reps.* Vol. xiv.
LEROQUE.—*Annals of Surg.* Nov. 1906.
LITTLEWOOD.—*Lancet*, Feb. 18, 1899.
FIRTH.—*Brit. Med. Jour.* 1882, Vol. ii. 166.

Chapter VIII.

ADHESIONS AND KINKING OF THE COLON.

ADHESIONS OF THE COLON.

Cases in which there are adhesions involving the colon are of considerable interest, for this condition is a not uncommon cause of severe constipation and abdominal pain, and occasionally even of acute obstruction. The condition commonly results in a severe degree of chronic invalidism, and as such merits close attention.

In some patients there are only a few adhesions, fixing or kinking the colon at one place, while in others the adhesions are extensive and general, involving the whole or a great part of the large bowel, and often the small intestine as well.

Where there is only a single band of adhesions, the condition is usually the result of some local inflammatory lesion such as an ulcer of the colon, inflamed glands, etc.; but where they are extensive it has arisen from a general peritonitis or from some previous operation or injury. Cases are met with, however, where no satisfactory explanation of the presence of adhesions can be found.

Baisch conducted some experiments upon animals to ascertain the cause of the formation of adhesions after operation. He did two series of experiments, in both of which similar peritoneal lesions were produced. In one series, complete hæmostasis was secured; in the other, varying quantities of blood were allowed to remain in the abdominal cavity. In the first series no adhesions developed, while in the second they were constantly present when the animals were killed.

When a patient recovers from general peritonitis, extensive adhesions between the different parts of the bowel and between these and the abdominal walls are undoubtedly left; but there is abundant evidence to show that in course of time these may entirely disappear. Numerous cases have been recorded, where the abdominal cavity has been subsequently opened either at an operation or post mortem (the patient having previously suffered from general septic peritonitis), and no trace of adhesions has been found. In some cases, however, the adhesions do remain after recovery from general peritonitis, and may cause serious consequences.

Why adhesions should remain in some cases and not in others cannot be explained until we know much more than at present as to the exact physiological processes which occur in the abdomen during recovery from peritonitis.

Some of the worst cases of general adhesions are those in which the condition has followed an operation upon the abdomen, and in which, apparently, the wound remained aseptic. Here it is probable that the result is due to blood having been left in the abdominal cavity. Extensive adhesions involving the transverse colon may result from a gastric ulcer, and the following case was probably of this nature :—

Case.—Mrs. R. was under my care in St. Mark's Hospital. She was sent to me by her doctor on account of repeated attacks of chronic obstruction, accompanied by severe abdominal pain and symptoms of chronic colitis. These symptoms had persisted for about four years, and in spite of treatment the attacks were becoming more severe and frequent. It was thought probable that she had some obstructing lesion of the colon, and an exploratory laparotomy was decided upon. On opening the abdomen, I discovered most extensive adhesions attaching the stomach and transverse colon to the anterior abdominal wall. The adhesions were so tough that they could not be separated, and I performed appendicostomy with the object of preventing accumulation in the colon, and so relieving her symptoms. It seemed probable that the condition had resulted from a perforated gastric ulcer some years previously, which had produced a local peritonitis. Subsequent enquiry elicited a history supporting this view. As a result of the operation there have been no further attacks of partial obstruction, but she still suffers at times from abdominal pain and discomfort.

Symptoms.

The symptoms produced by adhesions of the colon are numerous and varied. The most common are abdominal pain and discomfort, and chronic difficulty in getting the bowels to act.

The pain is often of a most indefinite character, and, although seldom severe, is usually more or less constant. It is worse when standing or walking, and is relieved by lying down. The patient often refers the pain to one or more definite spots on the abdominal wall, but these do not necessarily correspond to the situation of the lesion. The pain may be described as a chronic dragging pain, or as a dull colicky pain; it may be referred to the spine or sacral region. In some cases there is no actual pain, but a constant sense of discomfort in the abdomen, only relieved by lying down. Chronic constipation of a severe character is almost always present. The bowels only act as the result of using aperients or enemata, and even then often not satisfactorily, or intermittently.

Many sufferers from this condition become markedly neurotic, and it is a common cause of chronic invalidism. As a result

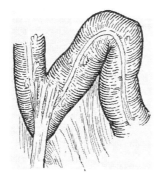

Fig. 33.—Kinking of pelvic colon from a band of adhesions.

of the constipation, they suffer from auto-intoxication, their complexion is bad, they have constant headache and neuralgia, the appetite is poor, and they lose weight.

In some cases there are recurring attacks of partial obstruction, with severe abdominal colic, and sometimes vomiting. After the administration of aperients and enemata the attack terminates with an action of the bowels, but is followed in the course of a few weeks by another.

Many of the patients suffer from chronic colitis, and pass large quantities of mucus in the stools.

Walking, or any form of exercise, increases the pain and discomfort; consequently the patient gets no exercise, and often not enough fresh air; as a result anæmia often supervenes.

The symptoms may persist for years, the patient occasionally getting temporary relief as the result of some new treatment, only to relapse again in the course of a few weeks or months.

If the adhesions are in the pelvic region there may be pain on micturition. If about the colon, they may cause pain by being dragged upon or stretched, or chronic obstructive symptoms owing to their preventing free movement of the bowel and giving rise to sharp corners and angles.

CHRONIC OBSTRUCTION FROM ANGULATION OR KINKING OF THE COLON.

From the existing literature on the subject, this condition would not appear to be very common, but it is probably more frequent than is generally supposed, and a not uncommon cause of some of the most serious cases of constipation. It is really the same thing as chronic volvulus, and cases described as chronic volvulus would be more correctly placed in this category.

In these cases there is an acute angle, kink, or twist in some portion of the colon, usually in the sigmoid flexure, which, though it does not entirely block the bowel lumen, constricts it to such an extent as to cause chronic obstruction to the passage of the intestinal contents, or causes the frequent impaction of solid fæcal material at this point, with consequent recurring attacks of more or less complete obstruction.

There is good reason to think that many cases of so-called congenital dilatation of the colon are due to kinking of the bowel from an abnormal mesentery; but the fact that the typical enormous dilatation and hypertrophy of the colon which is here present is not usually seen in cases of kinking, of which a considerable number, well authenticated, have now been reported, is opposed to such a view.

It is only comparatively recently that kinking has been recognized as a cause of chronic obstruction. Most of the earliest cases were described by Americans—notably by Tuttle, Delatour, and Leroque; but similar cases had been previously described in England under the title of "chronic volvulus of the sigmoid flexure."

One of the commonest situations for kinking to occur is at the junction of the mobile pelvic colon with the fixed upper end of the rectum. The apex of the pelvic loop is also a not uncommon situation.

OF THE COLON

Tuttle maintains that this condition of acute angulation may result from a congenital defect in the formation of the sigmoid mesentery, its line of attachment being too short and resulting in excessive angles at the extremities of the pelvic loop. There is, however, little or no proof of this contention.

The condition may result from any of the following causes:—

1. Contractions or adhesions in the mesosigmoid from inflammation.
2. Adhesions between two adjacent portions of the pelvic colon or between this and some other structure.
3. Abnormal length of the mesosigmoid.
4. Recurring volvulus.

Any inflammatory process which results in the formation of a local cicatrix or contraction in the mesosigmoid may result

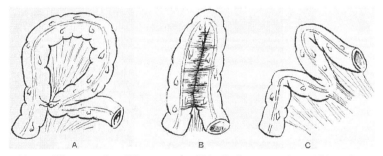

Fig. 34.—Diagram to show different ways in which adhesions may produce a kink or obstruction. (A) Two appendices epiploicæ adherent to one another. (B) The two sides of a loop adherent to one another. (C) A double kink caused by a band of adhesions.

in the formation of an acute kink or angle in the pelvic colon. Such a condition may arise from a caseating tuberculous gland in the base of the mesentery, from a diverticulum, from an abscess behind the peritoneum, and from such conditions as perimetritis.

I have operated in three cases in which the kink was found to be due to a broad band of peritoneal adhesion between the pelvic colon and the left iliac fossa. The peritoneal band formed part of the mesentery on the outer side, and was not separated from it. It was shorter than the mesentery itself, and in consequence an acute and abnormal angle or flexure was produced in the centre of the pelvic colon. In each of these cases the patient for several years had had difficulty in getting the bowels to act properly. In one case there had for some years been frequent and severe attacks of pain and obstruction, and in two others there was a history of severe and intractable constipation for several years. In all, the bowel trouble disappeared after division of the band. In none of them was any definite cause found for the formation of the band.

One of the commonest causes is undoubtedly chronic ulceration of the pelvic colon and pericolitis, with the consequent formation of adhesions between the peritoneum covering the base of the ulcer and some adjacent structure, the subsequent contraction of the adhesions producing a kink. Or two contiguous portions of the pelvic colon may become stuck together, with the result that an acute angle is formed at the apex of the loop. In one instance recorded by Tuttle, two appendices epiploicæ on

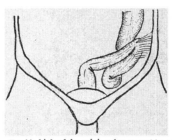

Fig. 35.—Double kink of the pelvic colon caused by adhesions.

contiguous portions of the pelvic colon had become adherent at their tips, thus forming a band which tied the loop together in the centre and constricted it.

In quite a number of the cases, appendicitis has been the cause. The sigmoid flexure has become adherent to the appendix or cæcum on the right side of the pelvis, and the weight of the proximal loop of the pelvic colon has resulted in an acute angle being formed at the point of the adherence on the right side, while in a few instances the appendix is found stretching across the pelvis, adherent at its tip to the sigmoid, and kinking it.

The condition may result from extensive pelvic adhesions following general or pelvic peritonitis. This is well known, and numerous instances have been met with. In such cases

OF THE COLON

the pelvic colon may be bent into several acute angles and much contorted, so that it is surprising that the fæcal contents are able to pass along it at all.

In one case (*Fig.* 35) two acute angles in the pelvic colon had arisen from extensive adhesions between the sigmoid and the vertebral column, the result of general peritonitis. Adhesions between the ovary or tubes and the sigmoid may cause a kink in a similar manner.

One would expect that dilatation and hypertrophy of the bowel above the obstruction would occur : this is so, but not to any marked degree. In one case, the bowel was ulcerated both above and below the constricted point, but it was doubtful if this was true stercoral ulceration. In several others, attacks

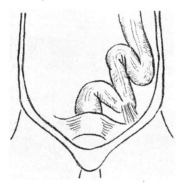

Fig. 36.—Angulation of the pelvic colon caused by adhesions to the iliac fossa. The condition produced chronic obstruction. (*Author's case*).

of diarrhœa would seem to indicate inflammation above the stricture. Fæcal impaction, and the formation of stercoral calculi in the colon above the constricting angle, have been present in several instances. The bowels will not act in these circumstances without the use of strong aperients, often aided by enemata administered with a long tube.

The condition does not appear to be fatal, except occasionally when fæcal impaction has occurred. Most of what is known about it is the result of what has been seen at operations done with the object of relieving the symptoms of chronic obstruction, aided by examinations of the bowel with the sigmoidoscope. Several times it has been possible to diagnose the condition by a sigmoidoscopic examination, and subsequent operation has confirmed the diagnosis. Normally, the pelvic colon will straighten out when the sigmoidoscope is pasesd, but where kinking exists, an abnormal fixed angle is seen which cannot be straightened.

There have been several instances in which a patient has been operated upon for intestinal obstruction, and on opening the abdomen, no obstruction has been discovered. Several cases have also been recorded in which acute obstruction was relieved by making an artificial anus above the distended coils of large bowel, and, after the obstruction had thus been relieved, the bowels commenced to act by the natural channel. In one case the patient died from an operation to close the artificial anus, and at the post-mortem examination no cause for the obstruction could be found. In another, the patient developed a ventral hernia in the scar of the first operation, and at the second operation, which was undertaken to remedy this, a careful exploration of the colon was made to find the cause of the previous obstruction, but nothing was discovered.

These are probably cases of acute angulation of the colon causing partial obstruction to the bowel lumen—in all of them there was a history of repeated attacks of partial obstruction and abdominal pain—the acute obstruction resulting from the colon becoming distended with fæces and gas. Distention would further accentuate the angulation or kink, and prevent anything from passing along the lumen. When the distention was relieved by colotomy, the kink was able to untwist, and the lumen again became patent. A careful examination of the mesosigmoid in similar cases will probably reveal that it is unduly long, or otherwise deformed.

The following case well illustrates this condition of kinking of the pelvic colon :—

Case.—Mr. I——, a gentleman aged 25, was brought to me by Dr. Leonard Williams on account of severe chronic constipation. He had suffered from this condition for three or four years. Every kind of non-operative treatment had been carefully tried, but he was no better and was anxious to have something further done. A sigmoidoscopic examination revealed a kink in the pelvic colon and fixation to the left iliac fossa.

On opening his abdomen a band of adhesions was found binding down the middle of the pelvic colon to the left iliac fossa and causing a sharp bend (*see Fig.* 36). The bowel was freed, and the peritoneum carefully closed in so as to leave no raw surface. He made a good recovery, and the bowels began to act regularly and without abdominal pain at once. When heard from six months later his bowels were acting regularly without aperients.

Favel reports a case in which a long mesentery to the cæcum and ascending colon was associated with severe pain in the abdomen. The patient was a woman, aged 32, who had suffered from several severe attacks of pain thought to be due to appendicitis. The appendix was removed and found, on microscopic examination, to be ulcerated, but there was no relief from the pain. A second operation revealed the fact that there was a long mesentery to the cæcum and ascending colon, with a band of adhesions fixing the ascending colon to the abdominal wall. The whole cæcal angle tended to revolve around this band and become twisted. The band was divided and the outer wall of the cæcum anchored by sutures to the iliac fossa. This cured the patient.

Paul Lercque records a case in which colitis and severe constipation were caused by shortening of the mesosigmoid by adhesions. Division of the adhesions resulted in a cure of the condition.

I have been able to collect twenty-four cases of angulation or kinking of the colon causing severe chronic constipation or complete obstruction, and in which the condition was verified by operation or post mortem. There can be little doubt that many bad cases of chronic constipation which are not infrequently met with are due to this cause.

Unless angulation is suspected and carefully sought for, it may easily be overlooked, even at an operation, when the abdomen is explored. The kink often occurs only when the patient is standing, and the force of gravity can pull down the pelvic colon into the pelvis. When the patient is recumbent, as he naturally will be during the operation, no kink may be seen. The condition, however, will not easily be missed if the pelvic colon is carefully examined for the presence of adhesions, the length of its mesentery, and the facility with which it can be kinked at its fixed ends.

Obstruction may result from a portion of the omentum being caught in a hernial sac, or in an operation scar, in such a way as to kink the transverse colon and obstruct the lumen. I once saw a case where a patient died from acute obstruction due to this cause : he was suffering from cancer of the rectum, and a left inguinal colotomy had been performed. The colotomy opening did not act, and five days after the operation the patient had developed all the symptoms of intestinal obstruction. On opening the abdomen, it was discovered that a piece of the great omentum had been taken up in the spur stitch in performing the colotomy ; this had caused an acute angle in the centre of the transverse colon, which had completely blocked the lumen. Clark has recorded a similar case, in which acute obstruction resulted from the omentum becoming adherent in a left inguinal hernia. The patient was successfully operated upon.

Adhesions between the gall-bladder and the hepatic flexure of the colon may cause obstruction. A case is recorded by Voelcker, in which the fundus of the gall-bladder had ulcerated into the colon.

Treatment.

Non-Operative Treatment.—While much can be done by non-operative methods to prevent the formation of adhesions after operations or an attack of peritonitis, they often fail when the condition has once become well established. When abdominal pain and discomfort are the chief symptoms complained of, a thorough trial should be given to non-operative methods before proceeding to perform laparotomy. In those cases where there are recurring attacks of obstruction, palliative measures seldom do any good, and operation is often the only method of relieving the symptoms.

It is usually impossible to tell how much benefit will result from careful medical treatment, and it is therefore always advisable, unless serious symptoms are threatening, to try the effect of massage and exercises, before proceeding to perform laparotomy.

Much can often be done by properly applied massage. For this to be effective, however, it must be well done, and combined with other forms of treatment. Too often the patient is told that he is to have massage, and is allowed to continue his usual mode of life, and the masseur simply comes in for half an hour a few times a week. In these days also, when almost every nurse considers herself a skilled masseuse, sufficient care is not taken to see that really skilled massage is being given. Such treatment is generally useless. The patients should for preference be in some nursing-home or institution where they can be kept under observation, and where proper electrical and vibratory apparatus is at hand. A really skilled masseuse is essential, and abdominal massage should be commenced gently. At first the patient should be massaged for not more than ten minutes, twice a day. This is much better than for twenty minutes once a day, and it will not cause so much fatigue.

When possible, the massage should be combined with electrical treatment. The sinusoidal current applied to the abdomen appears to be the most useful. The instrument should be capable of giving a quick break, and the current should be applied for about ten minutes at a time. High-frequency currents also seem to do good in some cases, but it is essential that the apparatus should be a good one, and not one of the toys so often seen in so-called electrical institutes.

The electrical application should be given first, and should be followed by massage. As the patient grows accustomed to the treatment, the period may be extended, but fifteen minutes' massage is usually sufficient, except in patients with very rigid abdominal walls. After the first week, exercises against resistance should follow the massage. These exercises should be those which contract the abdominal muscle and which flex the spine and thigh. Such exercises do good by moving the parietal peritoneum through the agency of the muscles in contact with it.

Treatment should be continuous at first, and the shortest time for a course which will do any real good is from a month to six weeks. During this period the patient should not be kept in bed, except, perhaps, during the first few days, but should be got out daily for a short time. After a course of treatment the patient should be instructed to take regular exercise, and to keep the bowels acting daily. The best forms of exercise are probably walking and riding. If marked improvement follows, the patient should have a second and shorter course of massage and electricity in about two months' time.

Injections of fibrolysin, a drug which is said to cause softening of adhesions, have also been used in these cases, and good results are claimed. The treatment is too new to warrant any opinion as to its benefit, but as the injections do not seem to cause any unpleasant results, the drug may be tried in conjunction with massage. The injections should be given intramuscularly, preferably into the buttocks, every two or three days.

In many cases, although some improvement follows a thorough course of massage, the patient soon relapses to the old condition, and in the worst cases little, if any, improvement occurs. Where a definite obstruction from kinking has occurred, nothing short of operation will do any good. Operation is indicated when there is serious difficulty in getting the bowels to act, and also when the patient is so greatly incapacitated by his symptoms as to prevent his attending to the ordinary affairs of life.

OPERATIVE TREATMENT.—The operation consists in separating or dividing adhesions and re-establishing the normal course of the bowel. Where only a few adhesions or a single band are present this may be an easy matter, but in other cases it may prove most difficult, either on account of the density and closeness of the adhesions, or because the bowel wall is friable from secondary ulceration. In one instance, at least, the bowel was ruptured in attempting to straighten it.

When the adhesions are very firm, or serious difficulty is experienced in straightening the bowel, the best procedure is probably to resect the involved loop and unite the ends of the bowel if this can be done, or to short-circuit the obstructing angle by lateral anastomosis.

It is not, however, sufficient merely to divide the adhesions in any case, since, if raw surfaces uncovered by peritoneum are left, the adhesions are almost certain to re-form and re-establish the original condition. The prevention of subsequent adhesions constitutes the chief difficulty in these cases. Various methods have been advocated by different surgeons, and various substances have been used to cover the raw surfaces with the object of preventing the formation of adhesions. Thus, painting over with gum or glucose has been tried. Covering them with gold leaf has been done a good deal, and with apparently good results. Filling the abdomen with salt solution, and subsequently giving large rectal or subcutaneous injections of water or salt solution, have been depended upon by some surgeons, while others again believe in abdominal massage and electricity applied to the abdomen for some time after operation.

None of these methods have been entirely successful in preventing the re-formation of adhesions, and there are numerous instances in which adhesions have re-formed after repeated operations.

Undoubtedly the best method is to bring the peritoneum carefully together, so as to cover all the raw surfaces left by division of the adhesions. This involves some form of plastic operation, and considerable care and patience. It is often possible, after dividing a peritoneal band transversely, to stitch the resulting wound in the peritoneum in a longitudinal direction, so as completely to cover in the raw surface, and at the same time straighten the bowel. The following is a good instance of the type of case which can only be treated satisfactorily by operation.

Case.—The patient, a married lady, was recently sent to me by her doctor. For ten years she had been a chronic invalid with mucous colitis. She suffered from a chronic pain in the abdomen, which at times became severe, and was always worst on the left side. She had lost weight, and always felt ill and depressed. She had fits of weeping and misery on the slightest, and often upon no, provocation, and was unable to go about or enjoy life in the ordinary way. She had an earthy complexion, and her appearance when I saw her was typical of toxæmia or auto-intoxication. Her stools contained large quantities of mucus, and often consisted of little else. A curious and unusual symptom was that the presence of anything in the rectum caused an uncontrollable desire to go to stool, and much tenesmus. She had been under medical treatment for years, and all the recognized non-operative measures had been tried. On examining the bowel with the sigmoidoscope, I found the mucosa quite normal in appearance. In the middle of the sigmoid, however, the bowel was firmly fixed and angulated, apparently by adhesions. The uterus was also found to be markedly retroflexed. It seemed probable that the tenesmus from which she suffered was due to the condition of the uterus, and a gynæcologist who saw her with me confirmed this view. I opened the abdomen and found a number of firm adhesions binding down and kinking the middle of the sigmoid flexure; these were divided, and the wound left in the peritoneum sewn up. The uterus was also drawn forward and anchored to the abdominal wall, so as to correct the position. The patient made a good recovery, and all her symptoms have now completely disappeared. When I last saw her, some months after the operation, she had put on weight, her complexion was good, she no longer had any mucus in the stools, and she told me she never remembered feeling so well and fit.

By similar means, and by utilizing loose folds of peritoneum, appendices epiploicæ, or omentum to cover in defects in the peritoneum, much may be done to prevent the recurrence of adhesions. Absolute ascepticity, and great care in removing all blood-clot from the peritoneal cavity, are, however, the most important factors in preventing their formation; and a subsequent course of massage and electricity is advisable.

The actual details of operation must vary with every case.

Many of the operations which aim at relieving obstructive angulation of the colon or chronic volvulus, by fixation of the bowel with sutures, fail to cure the condition. The patient is usually much improved, or apparently cured, immediately after the operation; but some months later the old condition comes back, and the constipation and chronic obstruction are soon as bad as ever. If a subsequent operation is performed, it is found that the adhesions have all given way and allowed the bowel to resume its previously abnormal position.

This seems to occur no matter what method of fixation is adopted, or how carefully it is performed, and it therefore seems as if the best operation in such cases would be to resect the affected loop of colon, or at least some part of it. This will effectually prevent recurrence by making the sigmoid a straight tube. This operation was adopted by Mr. Moynihan with success in one case after fixation had failed.

REFERENCES.

BAISCH.—*Beiträge zur Gebeits.* 1905, p. 435.
DELATOUR.—*Annals of Surg.* Nov. 1905.
TUTTLE.—*N.Y. Med. Journ.* March, 1908.
LEROQUE.—*Annals of Surg.* Nov. 1906.

CHAPTER IX.

ENTEROPTOSIS OF THE TRANSVERSE COLON AND HERNIA OF THE COLON.

ENTEROPTOSIS OF THE TRANSVERSE COLON.

ENTEROPTOSIS is undoubtedly an important causal factor in many cases of bad chronic constipation and in chronic mucous colitis. It is necessary to distinguish between true cases of visceroptosis due to the abdominal organs falling towards the pelvis, and those in which the apex of the transverse colon is dragged down and fixed in the pelvis by adhesions resulting either from a previous peritonitis or, less frequently, from adhesions to the neck of an old hernia. These latter cases are often incorrectly described as enteroptosis.

In extreme visceroptosis the centre of the transverse colon may lie behind the bladder, and I have seen two cases in which it lay in Douglas' pouch, and the lower border of the stomach lay behind the symphysis pubis. It is not uncommon to find the centre of the transverse colon as low as the brim of the pelvis. The transverse colon becomes longer from stretching, and often somewhat dilated. The splenic and hepatic angles are to some extent dragged down with the transverse colon, and thus come to occupy a lower position, while the angle formed at the two flexures is considerably more acute than in the normal condition. The normal position of the centre of the transverse colon is at about the level of the umbilicus or a little below this; but in complete enteroptosis the centre of the transverse colon becomes a pelvic organ.

Prolapse of the transverse colon cannot occur without gastroptosis, the relative positions of these two portions of the alimentary tract remaining much as before. In fact, enteroptosis of the colon only occurs as part of a general visceroptosis in which the colon, stomach, spleen, liver, and often the kidneys, are all involved. The diaphragm descends, and the peritoneal connections normally supporting these structures stretch and elongate.

Much importance has been attached to the increased angles or kinks at the hepatic and splenic angles of the colon which are produced in visceroptosis, especially with regard to their causing obstruction and chronic constipation. It seems doubtful, however, whether any serious obstruction to the bowel lumen is thus produced. If it were so, one would expect to meet with cases of acute obstruction from this cause, but I have been quite unable to find any unless complicated by adhesions. Dr. Hertz, who has studied visceroptosis under the

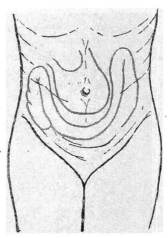

Fig. 37.—Diagram showing the position occupied by the stomach, and transverse colon in a bad case of visceroptosis.

X rays, has not seen any delay in the passage of the fæces past the flexures, such as might be expected to occur if there was obstruction of the lumen.

The chronic obstruction, or rather constipation, which undoubtedly does occur in cases of visceroptosis, is doubtless chiefly due to the sagging of the central portion of the transverse colon, which tends to the accumulation of fæces at this part, and to the fact that atony and weakness of the bowel musculature is generally an associated condition.

After visceroptosis has existed for some time, secondary changes occur in the transverse colon. The normal pouches or sacculations between the longtitudinal muscle-bands become larger, the whole bowel is stretched and more capacious, and the muscle coats atrophy. Chronic inflammatory changes in the mucous membrane, giving rise to the symptoms of mucous colitis, are common in such cases.

It seems certain that one of the most important factors—if not the most important—in visceroptosis is weakness of the abdominal muscles. The abdominal organs are kept in position chiefly by the positive pressure always present in the abdominal cavity from tonic contraction of the abdominal wall.

In visceroptosis the abdominal walls are usually weak and the muscles have wasted. Many of the secondary results of this condition must certainly be attributed to the venous stagnation in the abdominal vessels which occurs as the result of lowered intra-abdominal pressure.

Diagnosis.

Prolapse of the transverse colon can usually be diagnosed with certainty by means of the X rays, and the position of the stomach, which can be ascertained by palpation, is also a useful guide as to that of the transverse colon. Thus, if we find on palpation that the lower edge of the stomach comes down almost to the brim of the pelvis, we may assume that the centre of the transverse colon lies in the pelvis.

Treatment.

The patient often obtains much relief from wearing a properly fitting belt. This should come well down to the pelvic brim, and should support the abdominal wall in a direction towards the dorsal spine. If properly fitted, such a belt will, by restoring the intra-abdominal pressure, do much to relieve the worst symptoms. The object of the belt is not to act as a direct support to the stomach and colon, though this is often stated to be the case, but as an artificial abdominal wall, and thus to restore the intra-abdominal pressure which has been lowered by lax and badly-acting abdominal muscles.

In a normal individual the various abdominal organs are protected from the effects of gravity—which would otherwise tend to displace them all towards the pelvis—by the intra-abdominal pressure rather than by other factors.

Normally, the intra-abdominal pressure is sufficient to counteract the effects of gravity in the standing position, and the pressures on any intra-abdominal organ are practically equal in all directions, so that the slight anchoring supports which are provided by the various peritoneal connections are sufficient to retain the various organs in their correct relative positions. When, however, the abdominal walls become lax from any cause, the intra-abdominal pressure is lowered, and in some cases almost becomes negative, with the result that the organs in the upper part of the abdominal cavity are supported only by their peritoneal connections, which being quite inadequate soon yield, allowing the organs to prolapse. By means of a properly made belt, which should be worn always, except at night, the intra-abdominal pressure can be restored and the prolapsed organs will again be able to function properly. Much can also be done in some cases to develop the abdominal muscles by suitable exercises.

Many operations have been done with the object of relieving the chronic obstruction to the passage of the faecal contents along the bowel which results from prolapse of the transverse colon. Very careful consideration is, however, necessary before deciding upon such operations. It is obviously impossible to replace the transverse colon in its normal position, and secure it, without also fixing the stomach, and any operation which will entail a large abdominal incision or cutting the muscles transversely will tend rather to increase than diminish the tendency to visceroptosis, by weakening the abdominal wall.

The operations which have been performed are as follows :—

1. Suspension of the transverse colon by suturing the omentum to the abdominal wall high up.

2. Shortening of the gastric ligaments.

3. Repair of the abdominal wall (if damaged as the result of child-birth, etc.).

4. Excision of the whole colon.

Operations which aim at suspension of the prolapsed bowel are unsound in theory and almost invariably fail. It is hardly to be expected, when the normal suspensory ligaments have failed to support the bowel against a lowered intra-abdominal tension, that artificial ones will do so. Repair of the abdominal wall, in cases where the recti have become separated, is a sound operation, and will do good in suitable cases.

Surgical operations have often been performed for this condition, but they afford no certainty of relief, and by damaging the abdominal wall may make matters worse. They should not be done unless medical treatment has been well tried and has quite failed to ameliorate the symptoms, and unless their severity justifies an often dangerous operation, the result of which is more than doubtful.

HERNIA OF THE COLON.

Hernia of the colon is an uncommon condition, as from its position at the back of the abdomen the colon is prevented from reaching the hernial orifices, even should its mobility be sufficient.

Out of forty-seven cases of irreducible hernia collected from the records of St. Thomas's Hospital by Mr. Corner, the colon was found in the sac in only one.

But although this is one of the rare forms of hernia, it is of considerable interest, owing to the often unusual relationship between the bowel and its sac. The parts of the colon which may get into a hernial sac are those which possess a mesentery, either normally or as the result of some congenital abnormality of the peritoneum. Thus the cæcum, transverse colon, and pelvic colon may be found in hernial protrusions.

The cæcum, if it possesses a meso-cæcum, may find its way into one of the hernial openings. It is not uncommon in infants and young children to find the cæcum and appendix in a right inguinal hernia. This can also occur in the adult if the cæcum has a mesentery.

The cæcum may similarly find its way into a femoral hernia, and very rarely may be found in a left inguinal hernia. For the cæcum to be able to get into the latter, however, it must possess a very long mesentery, or a common mesentery with the small bowel.

Mr. Russel Rendle recently recorded a case in which the cæcum was found in a strangulated left inguinal hernia.* The patient was a male infant nine months old, who was admitted to the South Devon Hospital with a strangulated left inguinal hernia. At the operation, on opening the sac of the hernia, it was found to contain a loop of small bowel, and the cæcum

---

* *Lancet*, 1908, i. p. 1076.

and appendix. The hernia was reduced and a radical cure performed. The child recovered.

A case in which a left femoral hernia contained the cæcum is recorded in *St. Bartholomew's Hospital Reports*, vol. xxvii.

In cæcal hernia there is, as a rule, a complete sac, but occasionally, when the cæcum is found in a right inguinal hernia, it comes down behind the peritoneum and forms part of the wall of the sac.

The pelvic colon is also sometimes found in a hernial sac. If it has an abnormally long mesentery, it may become herniated in the same way as the small bowel. In this case there will be a complete sac. It may also be brought down into the wall of a large left inguinal hernia by the peritoneum being dragged

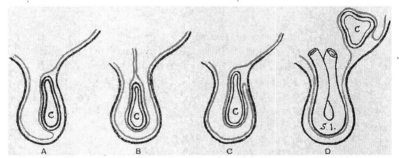

Fig. 38.—Diagram showing different forms of hernia of the colon :—(A) the colon forming part of the sac wall. (B) the colon completely inside the sac. (C) the colon partly inside the sac. (D) showing the manner in which the small intestine in a large left scrotal hernia may, by dragging on the parietal peritoneum, pull down the pelvic colon into the wall of the sac. The peritoneum is shown in red.

down to form the sac wall. This will only occur in the case of a large scrotal hernia, and the colon, under these circumstances, will be behind the peritoneum and will form part of the sac wall.

It may also occur as a congenital hernia owing to the peritoneum being dragged down to an abnormal extent in the descent of the left testicle. In this case the sac will either be absent or incomplete. A congenital hernia of the colon with a complete sac may occur, however, owing to the mesosigmoid being congenitally too long.

The transverse colon is not uncommonly found in a large umbilical or ventral hernia. It seldom gets strangulated, however, in such circumstances, though the writer has heard of two cases in which strangulation of the transverse colon occurred as the result of adhesions to the neck of an umbilical hernia. The transverse colon may also get into the sac of an inguinal or femoral hernia, and Mr. Paterson has recorded two cases of this condition.* In one, the transverse colon was found in a femoral, and the other in an inguinal hernia, both on the left side. Strangulation occurred in both cases. In order for this to be possible, the transverse colon must reach much lower than normal. The omentum gets into the hernia first and drags the colon after it.

In all cases of hernia of the colon, with the exception of cæcal hernia, strangulation is readily produced owing to the solid nature of the contents. Rarely the ascending or descending colon may be found in the sac of a lumbar hernia.

The chief importance of hernia of the colon is, that in those cases where the colon passes down outside the peritoneum and lies in the wall of the sac, great difficulty may be experienced in operating upon the hernia. Unless the condition is recognized, which is not easy, the bowel may be cut into, and in any case it may be difficult to return it into the abdomen.

The diagnosis of hernia of the colon as opposed to hernia of the small intestine is not possible apart from operation.

TREATMENT.

The treatment of a hernia containing the colon does not differ from that of an ordinary hernia containing small bowel, except when the colon forms part of the sac wall. There is a danger in such cases of cutting into the colon, or of including a portion of its wall in the ligature when tying off the sac.

If the surgeon is aware of the possibility of a hernia of the colon being present, he will usually be able to detect the condition when the sac is opened. Any adhesions should be most carefully divided, and the posterior part of the sac should not be separated, but returned, together with the bowel, into the abdominal cavity. In doing this, great care must be taken not to damage the blood-supply of the bowel. The deficiency in the peritoneum should be closed with stitches as carefully as possible.

---

* *Lancet*, 1908, vii. p. 237.

Chapter X.

INTUSSUSCEPTION.

INTUSSUSCEPTION is a condition in which one portion of the bowel, usually the upper, is invaginated into an adjacent portion. It may occur in any part of the alimentary canal, but in the majority of cases the lower portion of the ileum is invaginated into the colon (ileo-colic intussusception). The invagination may, however, be entirely confined to the colon (colic intussusception). It may involve a short portion of the colon or its entire length, so that the ileo-cæcal valve protrudes at the anus. There are many varieties of intussusception, depending upon the part of the bowel involved, the starting-point of invagination, and the number of layers entering and leaving the invaginated portion of bowel.

An intussusception may start in any portion of the colon, but it is always the upper portion which is invaginated into the lower. Retrograde intussusceptions do occur, but only during death or as the result of asphyxia; they are not met with in practice.

More than one intussusception may be present in the same patient, but such conditions are rare. Cases of intussusception involving the colon are usually divided into: (1) ileo-cæcal, (2) ileo-colic, (3) cæcal, (4) colic, and (5) appendicular. The subdivisions are not of much practical importance, as they merely depend upon the portion of bowel which originates the invagination, and the results of the condition are the same in all.

The commonest variety is the ileo-cæcal, in which the ileo-cæcal valve forms the apex of the invagination.

In some cases the intussusception becomes itself invaginated into the colon below it, thus producing a double intussusception. This condition may even be repeated, resulting in triple and quadruple intussusceptions.

As a rule the intussusception increases in length at the expense of the ensheathing layer, namely the colon. The apex remains the same, and as it is pushed forward by peristalsis, more and more of the sheath is drawn in to allow of its progression. The returning layer becomes creased and folded, so that it is usually considerably longer than the two others. There is only one exception to this method of growth of an intussusception, and that is in the ileo-colic variety, in which the ileum prolapses through the ileo-cæcal valve. As the condition progresses, more and more of the ileum prolapses, and the apex thus keeps changing, the intussusception growing entirely at the expense of the entering layer.

As the intussusception grows, the mesentery is dragged in between the entering and returning layer; as a result, the tumour becomes curved from the tension of the mesentery. Sooner or later the mesentery is strangulated, and, in consequence of its blood-supply being cut off, the bowel becomes gangrenous.

Etiology.

It seems probable that the normal occurrence of antiperistalsis in the cæcum and ascending colon has an important bearing upon the causation of intussusception. The most common form is that in which the ileum passes into the cæcum and colon, and it is obvious that antiperistalsis in the colon would tend to favour such a condition of things, as at one period in digestion there are two opposite waves of peristalsis occurring at the ileo-cæcal valve. The tendency would be for the smaller tube to become invaginated into the larger, and this is what occurs in intussusception. But since antiperistalsis of the colon is a normal condition occurring many times a day, and intussusception is a rare pathological condition, it is obvious that some other factors are necessary as exciting causes, though a predisposing cause normally exists.

There has within recent years been much speculation as to the causes of intussusception, and many most complicated explanations have been put forward.

In the hope of obtaining some positive information bearing upon the causes of this curious affection, I carried out a number of experiments upon cats. The animals were kept during the whole period of observation under an anæsthetic (ether). The influence of the anæsthetic to some extent interfered with the experiment; but as I was both unable and unwilling to carry out the experiments otherwise than under full anæsthesia, this had to be got over.

I found that if the animal was placed in a tank of warm saline solution before opening the abdomen, and if ernutin was previously injected, the anæsthesia did not seriously interfere with the movements of the bowel.

A small artificial intussusception was produced in the bowel by carefully invaginating a portion of the bowel into the part below it with forceps. In this way an intussusception in a downward direction and about 2 inches long was produced. The bowel was then left to see what would happen. In all cases the intussusception reduced itself in a period varying from ten to thirty minutes, the time depending upon the length of the intussusception. This was tried several times in different cats, but always with the same result.

The experiment was then tried of attempting to make the intussusception progressive by artificial stimulation of the bowel wall.

An intussusception some 2 to 3 inches long was produced as

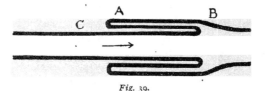

Fig. 39.

before, and a weak faradic current was applied to the ensheathing layer. The stimulus being applied at A in Fig. 39, the result was that the intussusception rapidly reduced itself.

When the stimulus was applied, a slight contraction occurred at the point of stimulation, but the strongest contraction was at the point B, opposite the apex of the intussusception; from there the contraction travelled backwards and reduced the invagination.

Stimulation of the entering layer at C produced the same effect, namely, strong retrograde contractions at B, with reduction. Wherever the stimulus was applied the effect was the same, namely reduction of the intussusception. It was not possible to make the intussusception progress by means of stimulation of the bowel wall; the effect was always the opposite, namely, rapid reduction.

Mechanical stimuli, by touching or nipping the bowel, were

INTUSSUSCEPTION

tried in place of the electrical stimulus, but the effect was the same. In some cases a slight contraction occurred at A, but within a few seconds, a second and stronger ring of contraction occurred at B, and passed backwards until the intussusception was reduced.

I then tried making an artificial retrograde intussusception in the colon; this soon reduced itself if left alone, and, if stimulated, reduced itself more quickly.

I found, in fact, that in a normal bowel wall an intussusception tended to reduce itself and not to be progressive, even when violent contraction occurred.

These experiments go to prove that an intussusception cannot occur in a normal bowel, but that some other factor must be present.

My experiments do not agree with those of Nothnagel, who said that he obtained artificial intussusceptions by tetanizing rabbits' intestine with electrodes. Experiments on the same lines carried out by myself have absolutely failed to produce a similar result.

The real explanation of intussusception seems to be clearly shown where a polypus is the starting-point of the invagination. The polypus acts as a foreign body and stimulates the bowel to pass it on; being attached to the bowel wall by a pedicle, it pulls this in after it, and, as the polypus is carried further and further down the bowel, more bowel wall is drawn in, and intussusception is produced. It seems probable that this is the real explanation in all cases. True, a polypus is not always present, but some other lesion is, which acts in the same way. Cases in which a polypus forms the apex of an intussusception are easily explained by this view, but it is not so easy to account for the common ileo-cæcal form met with in infants.

The late Mr. Barnard attempted this by assuming that prolapse of the ileum occurs through the ileo-cæcal valve, in the same way that prolapse of the rectum takes place through the anal sphincter. Prolapse of the rectum is common in children, and he believed that prolapse through the ileo-cæcal valve is also often present in children under similar conditions. He argued that the prolapse acts like a foreign body in originating the intussusception. There are, however, several facts opposed to this view.

Prolapse of the rectum usually occurs in children who have

INTUSSUSCEPTION

been neglected, who are thin, badly nourished, or recovering from illness, such as measles and whooping-cough, or it follows infantile diarrhœa.

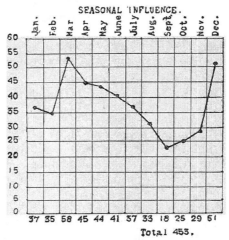

Fig. 40.—Chart showing seasonal incidence of intussusceptions in 453 cases not older than 12 months. (*Fitzwilliams.*)

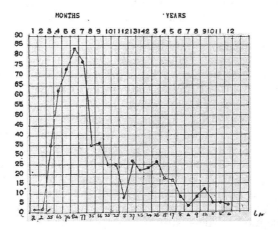

Fig. 41.—Chart showing age incidence in months and years in 648 cases under 12 years of age. (*Fitzwilliams.*)

Almost without exception, however, the infants who get intussusception are well nourished, fat, sturdy children, who,

INTUSSUSCEPTION

until the illness began, were in perfect health. Also, if intussusception resulted from prolapse, one would expect it to be common at those times of the year when diarrhœa is common, as is rectal prolapse in children. This is, however, far from being the case. Mr. Fitzwilliams, in a recent paper,* analysed 453 cases according to the time of the year at which they occurred. The chart (*Fig.* 40) shows that the condition is commonest during March and December, and least common in August and September, the months during which diarrhœa is commonest. Fitzwilliams has pointed out that March and December (owing to Easter and Christmas) are the times at which children are most likely to overeat themselves, or to eat indigestible foods.

While the prolapse theory does not seem tenable, the following explanation appears to be possible and to fit all the facts. If a

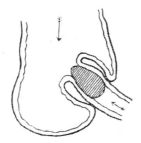

Fig. 42.—Diagram showing how a lump of indigestible food may produce an intussusception by becoming impacted in the ileo-cæcal valve.

child is given some indigestible food, part of this may form an indigestible bolus too large to pass through the ileo-cæcal valve. When it reaches this valve it either becomes impacted, or remains above and blocks it. Violent peristalsis will then occur in the ileum above, and the mass being unable to move, the whole ileo-cæcal valve is forced into the cæcum, the invagination being aided by antiperistalsis which is probably occurring in the ascending colon and cæcum as the result of food which has just previously passed the valve. Lumps of undigested matter are commonly found in the apex of an intussusception, and when they are not, it is reasonable to suppose that they have eventually become digested or have been squeezed through

---

* *Lancet*, February 29 and March 7, 1908.

the valve. This explanation fits in with the known incidence of the condition as shown by Fitzwilliams, and also with the fact that the ileo-cæcal variety of intussusception is so much the commonest.

Fitzwilliams suggests that the most probable cause of this condition in infants is the giving of unsuitable food before the child is able to digest it. Such food as crusts and biscuit are often given with the false idea of assisting the child to cut his teeth. There is every reason to believe this to be the correct explanation.

Cancer is not an uncommon cause of intussusception in the colon. The form of such a cancer is most commonly that in which the growth protrudes into the bowel lumen and forms a polypoid mass. The growth in such cases forms the apex of the invagination, and cases are on record in which a growth of the sigmoid or descending colon has projected at the anus. The late Mr. Barnard describes a form of intussusception which results from a relaxed or paralyzed condition of the colon, the healthy bowel invaginating into the relaxed portion. This condition usually leads to a chronic form of intussusception with chronic constipation rather than acute obstruction. Indeed, it is not improbable that some of the obscure and obstinate cases of chronic constipation result from a recurring intussusception of this nature.

The same observer also described a very rare form of intussusception of the colon which originated in gangrene of the transverse colon. The whole of the gangrenous portion of the colon was ultimately passed per anum, and the patient recovered, with a stenosis which required subsequent operation.

A case is reported by Mr. Ray,* in which an intussusception of the sigmoid flexure resulted from a subserous polypoid lipoma. The patient was a woman aged 30. The apex of the intussusception protruded from the anus. The patient was operated upon and the polypus successfully removed.

PATHOLOGY.

In acute intussusception, strangulation soon occurs and the invagination becomes irreducible. The blood-supply of the layers forming the intussusception is interferred with,

---

* *Lancet*, March 4, 1905

INTUSSUSCEPTION

and, as a result, there is œdema and swelling, which still further increases the strangulation of the intussusceptum or central portion. The sheath itself seldom suffers much damage, as its blood-supply is not interfered with; the chief mischief occurs in the middle layer.

The first serious change is that the entering and returning layers become firmly fixed together. This occurs first near the apex of the invagination,—that is to say, at the part which is the last to be reduced, the result being to make the intussusception irreducible. First, only the part near the apex is irreducible, but in time the whole may become so.

Later the two inner layers become gangrenous. This usually occurs first at the neck, where the collar formed by the turning over of the ensheathing layer constricts the entering layer. The time before gangrene may appear varies in different cases. It has been seen in thirty hours, but more usually it takes three to four days, and sometimes much longer.

Death as a rule occurs from exhaustion or peritonitis. The bowel above the intussusception does not usually undergo any marked alteration except in chronic cases.

In chronic cases of intussusception, there is obstruction but no strangulation. Even the obstruction is not complete, or at least is intermittent. If the condition exists for a long time, the usual secondary changes will be found in the bowel above, namely, dilatation and hypertrophy. Ulceration may also occur both in the intussusception and in the bowel above it.

Spontaneous Elimination of the Intussusception.—This occasionally occurs owing to gangrene at the neck allowing the invaginated portion of the bowel to become free, thus restoring the bowel lumen, and allowing the separated invagination to be passed per anum. As a result of the inflammation around the gangrenous area the entering layer and the sheath become fixed together, thus restoring the continuity of the bowel after the intussusception has been cast off. Very considerable lengths of bowel may in this way be eliminated, and cases are recorded in which as much as 3 feet or more of bowel have become separated and passed in the stools.

Spontaneous cure of an intussusception may thus occur, but it does not do so in more than about 1 per cent of cases, and recovery is doubtful even after it has occurred.

INTUSSUSCEPTION

Symptoms.

Intussusception may occur at any age, but is most common in early infancy. The late Mr. Barnard, from a study of 187 cases taken from the records of the London Hospital, found that 72 per cent occurred in children less than a year old, and 88 per cent in children under 10 years of age. Mr. Fitzwilliams, from an analysis of 648 cases occurring in children under 12 years of age, found that 72 per cent were in those under 12 months old; 20 per cent between the ages of 1 and 6 years; and 6 per cent between the ages of 7 and 12 years. He also found that the greatest number of cases occurred in infants between the 4th and 7th months of life.

The condition is much commoner in males than in females, the proportion being about 2 to 1. Fitzwilliams' statistics give 68 per cent males and 32 per cent females, figures which agree very closely with those of other observers.

Cases of intussusception divide themselves into two types: (1) Those in which the symptoms are acute; and (2) Chronic cases, in which symptoms persist for a considerable time without causing death.

Cases of the latter type are usually seen in adults, and in the common form of intussusception which occurs in infants the symptoms are almost without exception acute.

The symptoms in the acute cases are well marked and distinctive; and the following is typical of the variety most usually met with:—

The patient, a well-nourished and previously healthy infant, is suddenly seized with violent colic; it begins to scream, and shows all the signs of acute abdominal pain. It lies on its back with its knees drawn up, screaming with pain, and refuses to be pacified. The child usually vomits once or twice immediately after the onset of the pain. Though vomiting is a common occurrence at first, it usually does not continue, and is not a marked feature in most cases. There is much tenesmus and straining, and the child passes stools consisting principally, and sometimes entirely, of blood and mucus. The stools look like apple jelly, and are the most characteristic feature of the disease, and the one upon which the diagnosis principally depends. These apple-jelly stools are frequent, and their passage is accompanied by much straining. An examination of the abdomen reveals a distinct sausage-shaped tumour in about two-thirds of the cases. If the diagnosis is in doubt and nothing can be felt, an anæsthetic should be administered, when a tumour will usually be easily made out : it is sausage-shaped, and generally situated either in the right iliac fossa or across the abdomen at about the level of the umbilicus. In some cases the apex of the intussusception can be felt on making a rectal examination. The condition once established rapidly gets worse, and the child soon passes into a dangerous state, with collapse, coldness of the extremities, rapid pulse, and distended abdomen. If unrelieved, a fatal result generally follows in from two to eight days.

The typical symptoms are acute abdominal pain, coming on suddenly and accompanied by a palpable tumour in the abdomen, and blood and mucus in the stools. Such symptoms in a child are characteristic of intussusception, but although the clinical picture is as a rule well marked, considerable variations may occur. Thus the condition may supervene upon an attack of diarrhœa or indigestion, or the child may be seen before any stool containing blood has been passed.

If the child comes under observation soon after the onset of the illness, it may be difficult to make a correct diagnosis, though there will seldom be any doubt as to a serious abdominal lesion being present, and if the patient is watched for a few hours the diagnosis will be cleared up.

When the child is first seen after the condition has existed for some time, there will be marked collapse, with paleness and coldness of the extremities, the face will be drawn, the abdomen distended, and all the signs of impending death will be observed.

The diagnosis is generally not difficult. It depends principally upon being able to feel a tumour in the abdomen. This is a positive and certain sign. If there is doubt, and no tumour can be felt, an anæsthetic should be administered and the abdomen carefully examined bimanually with one finger in the rectum.

In the case of intussusception in adults, and chronic intussusception, the symptoms vary so greatly in different patients that it is impossible to give any characteristic symptoms or to lay down rules by which the condition may be diagnosed. The symptoms are those of intestinal obstruction coming on insidiously or of an intermittent character, and it is seldom that an exact diagnosis of the lesion can be made beyond the conclusion that some lesion is present, causing obstruction.

TREATMENT.

NON-OPERATIVE TREATMENT.—The proper treatment is immediate operation. Although reduction can sometimes be effected by the injection of fluid into the bowel per anum, this method is very uncertain. It only succeeds in a small percentage of cases, and reduction is often not complete. Failing the possibility of immediate operation, it should be attempted, but if an operation can be performed it is useless to delay operating while injection is being tried, for if the injection method fails, as it probably will, the patient will be in a less favourable condition for operation afterwards.

The Injection Method of Reduction.—The child should be anæsthetized, and placed in a position with the buttocks well raised on a cushion. A rectal tube is then introduced into the anus, and to this a glass funnel and tube are attached. Warm water is the best fluid, and this should be run in slowly with a drop of not more than about 3 feet. Gentle manipulation of the tumour through the abdominal wall will assist in reduction. The injection may need to be repeated before reduction is complete. If this is successfully accomplished, the child must be carefully watched for the next day or two to see that the intussusception does not recur, as it is apt to do.

OPERATIVE TREATMENT.—The abdomen should be opened near the middle line as a rule, but this will depend to some extent upon the variety of intussusception present, its position, and size. If the intussusception is not too large it should be delivered through the abdominal wound. If this is impossible owing to its size, it should be partly reduced in situ, and the remainder then delivered before reducing the last portion. The greatest difficulty is generally experienced in reducing the last two or three inches, and if possible it is advisable to be able to do this outside the abdomen, when the exact condition of affairs can be seen and the condition of the bowel better observed.

The best method of reduction is by catching hold of the colon opposite the apex of the intussusception and gradually squeezing the latter back. It is better if possible to avoid pulling upon the entering layer, and to reduce the condition entirely by squeezing back the apex of the invagination. In reducing the last two or three inches it is necessary to use the greatest care in order to avoid tearing the gut, which is often very friable at this point.

INTUSSUSCEPTION

If the condition can be completely reduced, and the gut is not too much injured to recover, the bowel should be returned into the abdomen and the latter closed as quickly as possible.

Intussusception usually occurs in very young children, and success depends very largely upon operating rapidly, and getting the small patient back to bed with as little delay as possible. For the first few hours the foot of the bed should be raised on blocks. Care should also be taken to see that the child's respiration is not embarrassed by heavy bedclothes resting upon the chest, since the breathing is already to some extent interfered with by the abdominal binder. Nourishment should also be administered as soon as possible, either by the mouth or rectum.

When reduction is not possible, or the bowel is too much damaged for there to be any reasonable hope of its recovery, it becomes necessary to consider what is to be done. The ideal method is to excise that portion of bowel containing the intussusception and to anastamose the ends. The difficulty is that in most cases the patient is not in a condition to stand so severe and prolonged an operation as this necessitates.

The only other alternative is to perform colotomy, either by excising the intussusception and tying a Paul's tube into the two ends of the bowel, or by bringing out that part of the intussusception which cannot be reduced, and after stitching it to the skin, opening it.

Much will depend upon the circumstances of the case and the skill of the operator. Except in adults and older children, most cases of irreducible intussusception die, whatever is done. There have, however, been several successful operations recorded in which resection and end-to-end anastomosis have been followed by recovery.

The following case recorded by F. W. Collinson[*] is a good instance of recovery after resection.

Case.—The patient was 3 months old. Symptoms of intussusception had been present for seventeen hours; chloroform was administered and the abdomen opened in the middle line. The intussusception was easily reduced, all but the last 4 inches, which were irreducible and dusky in colour. The bowel was clamped above and below, and the intussusception resected. The parts removed consisted of 2½ inches of the ileum, the cæcum, and part of the ascending colon, some 7 inches in all. The ends of the divided

---

[*] *Lancet*, October 19, 1907.

bowel were brought together with a Robson's bobbin and the abdomen closed. Two and a half hours after the operation the child was put to its mother's breast, and after this, feeding was continued every three hours. The bowels acted ten hours after operation. The bobbin was passed on the fifth day. The child made an uneventful recovery.

In chronic intussusception, operation is the only treatment. The greater part of the invagination is as a rule easily reduced, but there is often difficulty in reducing the last portion, and resection in some form has to be done. Resection with end-to-end anastomosis appears to give the best results and, owing to the better condition of the patient previous to operation, is not attended by so high a mortality as in the acute cases. The lower mortality from resection in chronic cases is also to some extent accounted for by the fact that the patients are generally older.

The following table shows the results of resection and end-to-end anastomosis by suture in 7 chronic cases of intussusception.

Czerny	F	age 36	Died.	
,,	M	,, 52	Recovered.	
,,	M	,, 13	Recovered.	
Boiffin	M	,, 24	Recovered.	
Braun	F	,, 23	Recovered.	
Müller	—	—	Died. N.B.—150 cms. resected.	
Rosenthall	F	,, 35	Recovered. N.B.—60 cms. resected.	

Prognosis.

This is good when operation is performed early and the intussusception can be reduced. It is bad in acute cases when more than twenty-four hours have elapsed since the onset of the condition, and when reduction is impossible.

References.

H. L. Barnard.—" Intestinal Obstruction," *Allbutt and Rolleston's System of Medicine*, 2nd ed. vol. iii.

C. D. L. Fitzwilliams.—" The Pathology and Etiology of Intussusception, from the Study of 1,000 Cases," *Lancet*, Feb. 29 and Mar. 7, 1908.

Chapter XI.

CHRONIC MUCOUS OR MEMBRANOUS COLITIS.

CHRONIC mucous or membranous colitis is a name given to a condition of which the chief symptoms are an excess of mucus in the stools, accompanied by abdominal pain, usually of a paroxysmal type. The condition is a badly defined one, and various names have been given it by different writers. To mention only a few : it has been described as colica mucosa, membranous or mucous diarrhœa, entero-colitis, mucous croup, enteritis membranacea, and glutinous diarrhœa. All these, and several others, have been used to designate what is without doubt the same complaint.

The distinguishing feature of the condition is the passage in the stools of mucus in abnormal quantities. Patients in whose stools this mucus is present, usually suffer more or less continuously from abdominal discomfort, from constipation which is often extreme, and occasionally in the more severe cases, from violent colicky abdominal pain.

This gives the essential features of a condition which has been described as a disease under the before-mentioned names, and about which much has been written. In Germany especially, long theses have been written upon it, and numerous speculations have been made as to its causation. Prof. Nothnagel, who was one of the first to describe it, believes it to be a secretory neurosis without any lesion in the colon, due to some condition of the central nervous system. He claims that the neurasthenia which often accompanies the disease is the cause of it. In this view Nothnagel has many followers, among whom may be mentioned Westphalen, King, Harrison, Osler, Weigert, and others. They get over the obvious difficulty that it is sometimes found associated with definite lesions of the colon, by putting these in a separate class and calling them secondary colitis. The condition has been compared to croup and asthma, and the most elaborate theories have been propounded to account for the various symptoms on the neurotic theory.

On the other hand, Von Noorden, Boas, Tuttle, the author, and other writers maintain that the condition is a real colitis, with definite lesions in the colon. The whole subject has become much confused, and the various hypotheses are so conflicting that it is difficult to unravel the truth.

The name itself is confusing, as colitis, if it means anything, implies inflammation, the existence of which many writers deny.

The condition has been variously classified and divided on every kind of basis ; thus we find one writer classifying the condition according to the appearance and form of the mucus present in the stools, while another divides it in reference to its supposed causes.

Symptoms.

Chronic mucous colitis is most frequently met with in women, between the ages of twenty-five and forty. It is, however, not uncommon in men, and one of the reasons why it is more frequently seen in women is that men are less prone to seek medical advice on account of vague symptoms, and consequently the less severe cases are often not diagnosed. Though it is most common between the ages of twenty-five and forty, it is by no means confined to this period of life ; several cases have been recorded in children ten years of age, and I have seen it in a patient of eighty-two.

The most characteristic symptom of the condition is the passage of mucus in the stools, and it is this which provides its name and often first draws attention to it. The mucus may be present in the form of shreds, or may form large casts of the bowel. I have seen such casts over a foot long, and the patient on seeing the casts under such circumstances is often much alarmed, not infrequently imagining that she has passed some curious and abnormally large worm. The amount of mucus present in the stools is often considerable, and they sometimes consist of little else.

In a typical case the symptoms occur periodically. Previous to an attack there is usually a period of constipation, the bowels for some weeks becoming more and more difficult to relieve. This is followed by a sudden paroxysm of acute abdominal pain. The patient feels ill, and has severe colic. In severe cases there may be vomiting, and a feeling of sickness is common. The pain continues with more or less severity for from twenty-four hours to a week. I have seen instances in which it was so severe as to necessitate the use of morphia, and to prevent sleep, and where the symptoms have been mistaken for intestinal obstruction or appendicitis. The temperature, however, is usually normal. The crisis terminates with an action of the bowels, most usually with diarrhœa. Each act of defæcation is, as a rule, accompanied by pain and tenesmus, so that the patient has been known to faint at stool. The first stools passed after an attack consist almost entirely of mucus, often in the form of casts or membranes. When the bowels act, the abdominal pain passes off and the patient is better for a time. In some patients the attacks recur as often as once a month, in others only twice or thrice a year. Some enjoy fair health in the intervals, while others are more or less chronic invalids. The paroxysms are most common in those patients who pass casts and large membranes, and it seems probable that the severe pain is due to the bowel becoming blocked by masses which have become detached from the mucous membrane, and to the violent peristaltic efforts at expulsion; it ceases as soon as the membrane has been got rid of.

Many patients with chronic mucous colitis, however, never have these attacks. They suffer from chronic abdominal discomfort rather than actual pain, and mucus is more or less constantly present in their stools. The tongue is furred, there is a feeling of discomfort after food, and great mental and general depression.

Flatulence and distention are common symptoms, and there is almost invariably severe constipation or a history of previous constipation.

The patient has generally a very poor appetite, often only being able to eat a few special articles of diet. One of my patients had practically lived on milk for eighteen months. As already mentioned, constipation is the rule. It is often severe, so that the patient is only able to relieve the bowels by large doses of aperients, and then at uncertain and infrequent intervals. In quite a number of cases, however, there is diarrhœa, though even in these there is an antecedent history of constipation. I have seen patients who had as many as sixteen and twenty stools in the twenty-four hours; but the diarrhœa is often to a large extent spurious; that is to say, there is very little fæcal material, but the stools consist of a small quantity, often not more than an ounce, of mucus and water. Therefore, although the bowels may be acting very frequently, the actual amount of fæcal material passed is often much below the normal. This diarrhœa is sometimes accompanied by considerable pain and tenesmus.

There is often considerable loss of flesh, and the patient is generally much below the normal weight. It is not uncommon for a patient to lose a couple of stone in the course of a few months. This loss of weight is perhaps best seen where there is diarrhœa.

Mental Condition.—This varies considerably. In a large percentage of cases the patient is markedly neurotic. She attaches quite undue importance to her condition, and can think of little else. Many are peevish and irritable : a trouble to themselves and to all about them. If, as is often the case, they have sufficient money to live a lazy life, they spend most of their time in bed or on the sofa, and in travelling to different health resorts. They never feel well or are comfortable, and to many of them life is a burden. They sleep badly, and can hardly get about at all. So marked is the neurotic element in many cases, that it is not surprising some observers have supposed it to be the cause of the condition. These cases form one of the worst classes of chronic invalids.

There are a number, however, in which the other symptoms are well marked, but the patients are not in the least neurotic. I have met with several such cases where the patient refused to give way to the symptoms, but got about as usual, and lived a busy and useful life. The condition is one which is naturally depressing, and it is no cause for wonder, therefore, when the patient is not obliged to work, the symptoms are allowed undue prominence, and neurosis and hypochondriasis occur. Examination of the abdomen, especially during an acute attack of pain, will often enable the colon—especially the descending colon and sigmoid—to be distinctly felt as a firm ridge. This is not because the colon is thickened, but because it is in a state of spasm, sometimes called enterospasm. If it could be seen, it would be found to be a firm tube with contracted walls.

The Stools.—The character of the mucus differs considerably in different patients, and also in the same patient at different times. It may appear as clear slime like uncooked white of egg, or as small clear lumps like tapioca. It may be present as whitish shreds, or strands, or in balls. Or again, it may occur in long tubular casts, either complete or broken up into strips. Sometimes it is passed almost in the pure state, while at others it is more or less mixed and discoloured with fæcal material. If these shreds are washed they can be seen to consist of laminated layers of pure mucin mixed with epithelial cells and food particles.

The stools are often pale in colour, owing to a deficiency in the secretion of bile. Blood is often present in small quantities, though it is necessary not to mistake blood from internal hæmorrhoids for that from the colon. I have found blood to be present in about 60 per cent of cases.

Intestinal sand is sometimes present. This curious material may exist in quite large quantities, and when first passed is of a reddish colour, almost exactly resembling ordinary sea sand, but afterwards becoming darker. One of the writer's patients passed as much as two ounces of sand in a day, but this is more than usual. In some patients it is always present in the stools, while in others it only occurs intermittently. Fæces containing this sand often cause considerable bleeding, from the scarifying action on the mucous membrane during their passage. Sand is generally only present in the more severe cases. In at least one case, the patient also passed uric acid gravel in the urine. The composition of this sand is approximately as follows :—Water 15 per cent, inorganic matter 51 per cent, organic matter 34 per cent. The inorganic residue contains salts of calcium, magnesium, phosphorus, iron, and also urobilin ; the chief inorganic constituent is calcium phosphate.

EXAMINATION OF THE PATIENT.—This should be thorough, and should include a careful examination of the stools on several different occasions; and, if possible, a specimen of fæcal material and some urine should be sent to a competent pathologist for examination and report. Special attention should be paid to seeing if there is blood in the stools. The amount of undigested food is also important, and if there is diarrhœa it is a good plan to give some charcoal with the breakfast on one or two occasions, and ascertain when this is first seen in the stools. The abdomen should be examined as regards the presence of tumours, thickening of the bowel, spasm, etc. Also the stomach should be percussed to ascertain whether any marked degree of visceroptosis exists. After this the patient should be made to stand up, and the abdomen be examined for weakness of the abdominal walls. The rectum should be examined, and a careful sigmoidoscopic search made to ascertain the condition of the pelvic colon. This last is essential; otherwise the diagnosis is little better than guesswork, and if a local lesion exists, as it usually does, it will almost certainly be missed.

PATHOLOGY AND ETIOLOGY.

Chronic mucous colitis is a condition the very name and description of which are based entirely upon its clinical symptoms, and it is very difficult to deal with such a condition upon a purely pathological basis. I trust, therefore, that I shall be in part excused for any confusion of terms or misapplication of names which may occur in the attempt here made to so deal with it.

Before going further it is necessary to consider Nothnagel's theory that the condition is a sensory neurosis.

The Neurosis Theory.—Nothnagel maintained that no pathological lesion in the colon could be found, but he was admittedly unable to see whether such a lesion was present or not, with the exception of a few cases in which the patient died from some intercurrent disease and a post-mortem examination was possible. In five such cases, which will be referred to later, no lesion of the colon was found in one, but a lesion was present in the remaining four. In four others in which a post-mortem examination was made upon patients who had suffered from mucous colitis at some period during their lives, no lesion was found. These cases were reported respectively by Rugez, Edwards, Osler, and Jagic. Thus, out of a total of nine cases in which a post-mortem examination was made, no lesion in the colon was found in five. It must also be taken into consideration that the condition is not itself fatal, and that several of the patients had not had symptoms of colitis for some time previous to death. Even as negative evidence this is not strong.

The other fact which Nothnagel made much of to support his theory was that most of the patients are neurotic. But typical cases of chronic mucous colitis occur in which there is no neurosis; on the other hand, we commonly see sufferers from chronic prolapsed piles or some similar ailment, who have become markedly neurotic, but we should not think of arguing that the piles were caused by the neurosis. It is evident that Nothnagel's theory with regard to the causation of chronic mucous colitis rests upon the slenderest evidence, and that of a purely negative character.

It is impossible to arrive at any satisfactory conclusion with regard to the pathology unless definite data as to the condition of the colon are obtainable. Until recently such data were only possible after a post-mortem examination following the death of the patient from some intercurrent disease. Lately, however, the surgeon has on many occasions been called to operate upon these cases, and an opportunity has thus been afforded of examining the colon during the progress of the operation. Also, within the last few years, the introduction of the electric sigmoidoscope has made it possible to examine the interior of the pelvic colon in such cases and to see the condition of its walls.

I have collected eighty cases of this condition in which data have been obtainable, and it is on this evidence that the statements here made are founded. Hitherto the cases of chronic mucous colitis collected by different writers have been taken indiscriminately, and in the majority of them there is no evidence whatever of the condition of the colon. This is true of the collected cases of Hale White, Von Noorden, and Harrison, and these series, though of value from the clinical aspect, are useless from the pathological.

In the series here given of 80 cases, only those have been taken in which either some lesion of the colon was found to be present, or in which such a lesion was more or less definitely excluded either by post-mortem examination or by operation.

CASES IN WHICH A POST-MORTEM EXAMINATION WAS MADE.

Rothmann	An inflammatory condition of the mucous membrane of the colon was found.
Abercrombie	There was a chronic cystic condition of the whole mucosa of the colon.
Hemmeter (2 cases).	A histological examination of the wall of the colon showed chronic inflammation of the mucosa.
Weigart. Osler. Edwards (2 cases). Jagic.	No pathological condition of the colon was discovered.

Of the cases which I have collected, I will take those first in which no cause for the condition was discovered. There are 14 such cases.

In four, no lesion was found, but blood was present in the stools in addition to the mucus. Now bleeding cannot occur without an abrasion of the mucous membrane or some pathological condition; it is therefore certain that some lesion did exist in the colon in these cases, though at the operation nothing abnormal was noticed.

In none of the remaining ten cases was the whole colon thoroughly examined, and they cannot, therefore, be taken as certain evidence that no lesion was present.

In all the other 66 cases a definite lesion was known to be present. The nature of the lesion varied considerably.

	CASES.
Adhesions and pericolitis causing more or less kinking and obstruction..	14
Enteroptosis of the colon ..	5
Chronic appendicitis	5
Inflammation or displacement of the uterus or appendages ..	2
Previous operations upon the abdomen and involving the colon	2
Chronic inflammation of the colon ..	30
Cancer ..	7
Fibrous stricture of sigmoid	1

In two cases there was old-pelvic cellulitis and the sigmoid flexure was involved in the adhesions. In one case an abscess had burst into the colon two years previously, and much thickening round the sigmoid flexure could be felt. There was also blood in the stools. One patient had had a previous attack of gall-stones, accompanied by local peritonitis in the neighbourhood of the gall-bladder.

In two, the colitis began after a severe attack of gastric ulcer from which the patient had recovered without operation. One of these patients, a woman, age 45, was subsequently operated upon, and extensive adhesions were found binding the stomach, great omentum, and transverse colon so firmly to the anterior abdominal wall, that they could not be separated without serious risk of tearing the bowel. One patient had had a large abscess in the back of the pelvis opened and drained through the abdominal wall, and the colitis dated from this. In three, the sigmoid flexure was found to be bound down and kinked by a band of adhesions.

In several of the cases there was definite thickening of the colic wall, or chronic inflammation of the mucosa, in addition to the adhesions.

The adhesions seem indirectly to cause the increased mucus and membrane in the stools by kinking or narrowing the colon. This results in the fæcal contents passing slowly, or being temporarily retarded, with consequent local irritation and inflammation of the mucosa.

Enteroptosis is only an indirect cause of colitis, and should rather be considered as giving rise to the constipation to which the colitis is secondary. Some of the worst cases of membranous colitis that I have seen, have been due to enteroptosis. Not only is the mesocolon lengthened, allowing the colon to fall into the lower part of the abdomen, but the colic wall itself shows well-marked changes: it is thinned and dilated, often to a considerable extent. The normal pouching is much increased, and the wall bulges between the longitudinal muscle-bands. If the interior of the sigmoid is examined with the sigmoidoscope, the walls can be seen to bulge inwards in such a way that they tend to prolapse into the part of the bowel immediately below.

In two of my cases, both women, the centre of the transverse colon lay in Douglas's pouch; and in one, the centre of the sigmoid flexure could reach the edge of the liver. As one would naturally suppose, severe constipation accompanied the condition.

Chronic Appendicitis.—There has been much discussion as to the relationship between this and chronic colitis. That the two conditions are frequently associated there can be no doubt. Colitis not uncommonly results from chronic inflammation of the appendix, or the two may occur together, the one complicating the other. There is very positive evidence that chronic appendicitis may cause colitis. Mr. Lockwood has recently recorded three cases of colitis in which the removal of a chronically inflamed appendix resulted at once in the disappearance of all the colitis symptoms; in each of the cases the appendix contained septic material which periodically escaped into the cæcum. In five of my collected cases, a chronically inflamed appendix was found, and its removal resulted in the disappearance of the colitis. In three of these, large mucous casts had previously been passed, and this is of interest, because some writers attempt to draw a distinction between mucous and membranous colitis.

A certain amount of colitis must almost invariably accompany chronic appendicitis, and as Lockwood has pointed out, it is common to find a certain amount of inflammation of the ascending colon when operating for appendicitis.

Chronic appendicitis can apparently give rise to colitis in three ways :—

1. By the inflammation spreading from the appendix directly to the cæcum, ascending colon, and transverse colon ; we have evidence of this in many cases of chronic appendicitis.

2. As a result of appendicitis, adhesions may form between

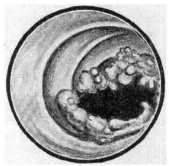

Fig. 43.—Malignant tumour in the sigmoid flexure, which gave rise to symptoms of colitis as seen and diagnosed by the sigmoidoscope.

the appendix or cæcum and other parts of the colon, usually the sigmoid. These adhesions, by constricting the lumen of the bowel, either directly or by the formation of kinks and abnormal angles, may result in a local inflammation of the mucosa, which spreads to other portions of the colon.

3. The inflamed appendix acts as a septic focus which is constantly discharging septic material into the colon. It seems as reasonable to consider this a cause of colitis as to consider gastric ulcer and gastritis a result of septic conditions of the mouth and teeth.

Malignant Disease.—In seven of the cases the colitis was found to be due to cancer in the colon. In all of them the growth was in the sigmoid flexure. In three the membranous casts supposed

PLATE III

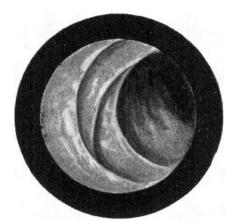

Fig. A.

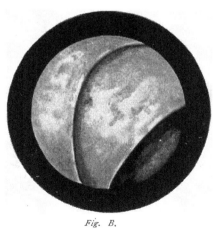

Fig. B.

CHRONIC COLITIS.—Sigmoidoscopic appearance of the pelvic colon in two cases.
(*Author*).

by some to be typical of the neurotic form of colitis were found in the stools. In all of these cases the condition had been diagnosed as chronic mucous colitis. In six, the growth was discovered on examining the bowel with the sigmoidoscope, and in one case appendicostomy was performed for supposed chronic colitis, the patient subsequently developing obstruction, which drew attention to a cancer of the sigmoid.

Chronic Inflammation of the Colon.—In thirty of the cases the cause was found to be a chronic inflammatory condition of the mucosa. In most of these the condition of the mucosa was directly examined by means of the sigmoidoscope. In all, a true colitis was present, but the type of inflammation differed.

Hypertrophic Colitis.—In this condition the mucous membrane is paler than normal, and considerably swollen, due to submucous œdema. The mucosa tends to lie in folds or concentric rings, and to prolapse into the lumen in a characteristic manner. The bowel wall appears to be redundant, and somewhat resembles a series of short intussusceptions at the part under observation. This condition is associated with excessive secretion of a thick glairy mucus, which can be seen sticking to the bowel wall in long bridges or loops. The reaction of this mucus is sometimes acid.

Granular Colitis.—This is present in a number of cases. The granular appearance of the mucosa is often very marked, and gives it a curious appearance as the light is reflected from each little swelling. This is due to inflammation of the follicles in the mucosa; each follicle is swollen, and projects above the general surface. The condition is a precursor of follicular ulcerative colitis, and it is not uncommon to find that some of the follicles have broken down and formed ulcers. The mucosa is inflamed and often of a dusky-red colour. In several of the cases in which I have been able at a subsequent operation to examine the bowel wall, I have found it much thickened, and in one there was also some enlargement of the lymphatic glands in the mesosigmoid. (See *Plate III.*)

Chronic Catarrhal Colitis.—For want of a better, this name must be used, as there is no particular feature to differentiate this form of inflammation. Here the whole visible mucous membrane can be seen to have lost its normal glistening appearance, and to be much redder than the normal mucosa. In a well-marked case the appearance is as if the surface had been rubbed off with sand-paper. The surface bleeds readily if touched, and apart from this, small bleeding areas can be seen. Here and there patches of yellow membrane-like mucus can be seen adhering tightly to the mucosa ; and if these are wiped off, the subjacent mucosa will bleed. The inflammation is not uniform, but is always best marked at the apices of the folds, and on the upper surfaces and edges of the valvulæ conniventes.

The appearance of the mucosa in cases of colitis bears a close and remarkable resemblance to the inflammatory conditions of the throat. I have seen the exact appearance of granular pharyngitis in the sigmoid flexure, and in many cases of colitis which I have examined, the appearance irresistibly reminded me of what is usually described as a septic sore throat. The condition of the mucosa in colitis varies much, even in the same case. At one time the mucosa will look almost normal, while at another the conditions described may be seen. The condition is a chronic one, but the degree of inflammation varies very much from time to time.

Though for purposes of description it is convenient to divide up the types of inflammation seen in colitis, it is not unusual to find more than one type present in the same case. Ulcers in the mucous membrane are also often seen in colitis, but they will be dealt with in considering ulcerative colitis.

From the statistics here given it seems safe to conclude that, in the great majority of cases of so-called chronic mucous or membranous colitis, a definite pathological cause for the symptoms exists, though these causes are of widely varying chaarcters in the different cases. B. V. Beck, in Germany, has come to a similar conclusion from the study of a large number of cases.

A careful study of the cases which I have collected, and of the pathological data obtainable in cases of chronic mucous or membranous colitis, leads inevitably to one conclusion, namely, that mucous and membranous colitis, as ordinarily described in text-books and medical treatises, is not a disease, and has no claim to be considered as a clinical entity. It is clearly a collection of symptoms which, from want of better knowledge as to the pathology of the colon, have been described as a disease, whereas in fact these symptoms may be due to many different pathological conditions of the colon, of widely different characters.

MEMBRANOUS COLITIS

The name mucous or membranous colitis should not be used, as it depends upon the presence of mucus in some form or other in the stools; and as I have already shown, there is excess of mucus in a great variety of different pathological states of the colon; and further, the form which the mucus takes, whether shreds, casts, or membrane, is of no real or pathological importance, membrane and casts being merely a rarer form in which the mucus may exist in the dejecta. (See *Chapter II.*)

The name chronic colitis should be retained, but should be used only to designate those cases already described in which a definite chronic inflammatory condition of the mucous membrane of the colon is known or supposed to be present.

The word colitis means inflammation of the colon, and is therefore correct as applied to those cases, but is not correct if the condition is a neurosis, or if due to pathological conditions not dependent upon inflammation.

Previous writers have argued that chronic colitis is a neurosis because in certain instances no lesion can be found in the colon, and it cannot be denied that there are such instances, though they are rare. It seems most reasonable to explain such cases as being those in which imperfect observation has failed to find the cause, which nevertheless did exist, rather than to assume that they are a special class in which there is no pathological lesion.

But even if we admit that cases occur without any pathological lesion in or around the colon being present, it is not correct to describe these as colitis, and they should not be included.

TREATMENT.

NON-OPERATIVE TREATMENT.—If the patient is seen during an attack, it will be necessary first to relieve the acute symptoms, and especially the pain, before proceeding to deal with the colitis. The indication is to empty the colon of the contained mucus. The plan I have found most satisfactory is to first give a hypodermic injection of morphia, in order to relieve the spasm and pain, and then to administer a large olive-oil enema. This should be given very slowly, with the patient in the left Sims position, and about a pint should be injected. At least fifteen minutes should be occupied in giving the enema, and when it is all in, the patient should assume the knee-elbow position for a few minutes to allow the oil to run well up into the colon. An hour or two later, a plain warm-water enema of about two pints should be given. This will generally result in bringing away the mucus, and will terminate the attack; if not, it should be repeated.

The non-operative treatment of chronic mucous colitis consists in getting the mucous membrane of the colon back into a normal state. For this purpose nothing seems better than injections of olive oil. The oil should not be used as an enema, but should be retained as long as possible, in order that it may act as a dressing to the inflamed mucous membrane. I order from a half to one pint of warm olive-oil to be injected very slowly into the rectum at bedtime. After assuming the knee-elbow position for a few minutes in order that the oil may get well up the colon, the patient should remain quite quiet and, if possible, retain the oil till next morning. If it is properly administered, most patients will easily retain half a pint, and I have known several who, after they had become accustomed to the injections, could retain a pint all night. Next morning a warm water enema is administered. Under this treatment the colitis often quickly clears up, and the mucous membrane soon assumes a healthy appearance. Sometimes it will be found that some stimulating application is needed, as the mucous membrane remains in a chronically inflamed condition in spite of the oil. The best injections under such circumstances are protargol or argyrol in ½ per cent solutions. Nitrate of silver should never be used, as it causes severe burning pain and does no more good than the albuminates of silver, which are painless.

When protargol is used, it should be given in place of the oil, and the bowel should first of all be washed out with warm water. The injections should be made with a No. 10 soft rubber catheter and a glass funnel, not with a syringe. It is most important in cases of chronic colitis to treat the constipation which almost invariably accompanies it. While the oil is being administered, the bowels will act without difficulty, however, and no aperients should be given.

Personally, I believe it is better not to administer aperients at all in cases of chronic colitis if they can possibly be avoided, as they help to keep up the condition. The best aperient is castor oil, if one has to be given. Dr. Hale White believes in treating colitis by half-ounce doses of castor oil administered on waking in the morning. The only other aperients which are allowable are sulphate of magnesia and small doses of cascara. Metallic aperients, such as calomel, should on no account be given, because they increase the inflammation of the mucosa and aggravate the disease.

Among the drugs which have been advocated for colitis, mention must be made of belladonna. This often has a good effect in preventing the spasm of the colon which is so common. The following antispasmodic mixture I have often found to do good in cases of colitis :—

℞	Tinct. Hyoscyami	..	..	℥ss
	Tinct. Belladonnæ	..	..	♏vj
	Sodæ Bicarb.	..	..	gr. xx
	Tinct. Zingiberis	..	..	♏xv
	Spt. Chloroformi	..	..	♏xx
	Aq. Menth. Pip.	..	..	ad.℥j

Misce. One ounce three times daily.

Arsenic in full doses is also recommended, and seems to do good in some cases.

Diet.—The old-fashioned treatment for chronic colitis was to feed the patients with milk and easily digested slop dietary, with the object of keeping the colon empty. This is a mistake ; the normal colon is never empty, and there is no object in trying to keep it so. Moreover, these patients require feeding up, in order that their general condition may improve, and it is most important they should be given a full diet. Von Noorden has, I think, proved that the old plan was a mistake ; and patients treated with his form of dietary certainly do much better, and the colitis clears up more quickly, than was the case with the old method.

Von Noorden's principle is to give a full diet containing an excess of indigestible residue : that is to say, cellulose and fibre. The patient should have plenty of vegetables and fruit, brown whole-meal bread in place of white bread, and a small amount of brown meat. The diet should be a full one, in fact as much as the patient can eat. The result is, of course, to cause copious fæces, owing to the large amount of indigestible material in the food. If such a diet were given alone, it would result in hard, firm stools, which it is particularly desirable to avoid : to get over this, therefore, a sufficient quantity of fats must be added to ensure the fæces not becoming formed. The alimentary canal can only absorb a very limited amount of fat, and if, therefore, an excess is given, the remainder will pass out in the fæces, and, as fats are liquid at body temperature, will prevent the fæces becoming hard, and keep them soft and unirritating.

The amount of fat required must be gauged by the stools, which should be about the consistency of ointment, and should be quite unformed when passed.

The fat is best given as butter, milk, fat bacon, and cream. The addition of about two ounces of thick Devonshire cream to the diet will in most cases produce the desired effect upon the stools. In some patients the excess of fat causes biliousness and indigestion, and on this account they are unable to continue taking it. When this is the case petroleum should be substituted for the fat. Petroleum, in the form of "Lenitol" (Rouse & Co.), or the liquid petroleum of the B.P., can easily be taken by the mouth, as it is quite tasteless, and beyond the greasy sensation is not unpleasant. This is not absorbed in its passage along the alimentary tract, and all passes out as it goes in. If the correct quantity is given, it absolutely prevents any solidification of the fæces. In most persons, three teaspoonfuls of "Lenitol" by the mouth in the 24 hours will render the fæces quite soft and unirritating, but the exact quantity required must be ascertained by experiment. Fat is, however, better than petroleum when it can be taken, as it helps the patient to increase his weight, which is very desirable in most cases.

The first effects of Von Noorden's diet are often to cause discomfort from flatulence and indigestion. In some, it may even cause nausea. This is hardly surprising, considering that the patient as a rule has been living for some time on a minimum of food, and has no appetite. These unpleasant symptoms, however, soon pass off; and he begins to see the benefit of the changed dietary. The weight rapidly increases, the bowels begin to act regularly, and there is a steady improvement in the general health. In order to overcome the initial discomforts which often result from the diet, and to prevent the patient giving up the treatment, it is advisable to keep him in bed at the beginning, and to order gentle abdominal massage. The massage should be for about ten minutes, an hour after each meal, and along the line of the colon. This will quite prevent any discomfort, and will greatly assist the action of the bowels.

MEMBRANOUS COLITIS

I have often seen patients, who for years had never had an unassisted action of the bowels, get two natural motions a day directly this treatment is adopted. As a rule they quickly get accustomed to the diet, and are able to dispense with massage in ten days or a fortnight : It should be continued for some considerable time, not stopped directly the symptoms disappear. No aperients should be allowed.

OPERATIVE TREATMENT.—This condition, like so many others, is one of those in which, purely medical treatment having failed to give relief, the aid of surgery has of recent years been called in.

Hale White has stated that in many cases a cure cannot be expected from medical treatment, and that in one-third no alleviation of the condition results from it. Beck goes further, and says that none of the cases treated medically are cured. While Beck certainly overstates the case, there is no doubt that in a considerable number of cases the surgeon is called in because medical treatment has failed to do any good. This failure must be to a considerable extent attributed to the fact that the cause of the condition has not been found, and that, in consequence, the appropriate treatment has not been adopted ; the first essential of treatment in these cases being a correct diagnosis as to the underlying cause of the symptoms. As I have already shown in discussing the pathology, the cause is in many cases one which can only be dealt with by surgical operation.

I shall here only discuss the treatment of cases of real chronic colitis (i.e., where an inflammatory condition of the colon exists), as in the others the treatment naturally comes under other headings, according to the pathological condition found, the obvious indication being to remove the cause whenever possible ; this may be a chronically inflamed appendix, adhesions, cancer, disease of the uterus or appendages, etc. In order to make a correct diagnosis, an exploratory laparotomy may be necessary, and in this case the operator will proceed to deal with whatever cause is found, or to do whatever operation he considers advisable.

The first published operation for chronic membranous colitis was done at the suggestion of Dr. Hale White by Mr. Golding Bird in 1895, though apparently the first operation performed for this condition was by Mr. Keith in 1894. In both the operation consisted in establishing an artificial anus on the right side, in order to deflect the fæcal current and give rest to the colon.

In considering the surgical treatment, we have to bear in mind that the condition is not a fatal one and in no way threatens life, but calls for treatment on account of the disablement and distress it causes. Surgery has attempted to cure the condition in two ways :—

1. By deflecting the fæcal current through the colon, so as to give the latter complete rest.

2. By establishing an opening through which the colon can be constantly washed out and kept clean.

Of these, the first was the method adopted in all the early cases operated upon. A right-sided colotomy or cæcostomy was performed, and the fæces thus prevented from passing along the diseased colon.

In the first case operated on by Mr. Golding Bird, the patient was much benefited by the operation. The colotomy opening was closed in seven weeks, and the patient appeared to be cured of her colitis. But five weeks later she died suddenly from peritonitis, the cause of which was not discovered.

I have found records of six cases in which an artificial anus was established on the right side, in five cases the cæcum being opened and in one a right lumbar colotomy being performed. In all these the symptoms rapidly and completely subsided after the colon was put at rest. In all of them the symptoms had been severe, and had resisted all other forms of treatment. The artificial anus was kept open for varying periods, from six weeks to three years. It was found that if the opening was closed too soon, the symptoms were liable to return.

In one of Mr. Golding Bird's cases the colotomy was closed in a year, and the patient remained well for six years from the original operation, but then relapsed. In two cases, the patient was quite well and had had no relapse four years after the operation; the others were well up to periods less than this. One died, as already mentioned.

As regards, therefore, a cure of the colitis, right inguinal colotomy or cæcostomy gives very good results, especially if the opening is maintained for some time; Hale White advises that it should be left open at least a year. The operation is, however, not a satisfactory one, and has been but little adopted. A right-sided colotomy is a most objectionable operation to the patient; the fæces are fluid and cannot be properly controlled, the skin becomes excoriated, and most patients would prefer the colitis to the discomforts which necessarily accompany such an operation.

The opening can be closed again, but must be left open for many months if it is to be of any use. The closure is not, moreover, always an easy matter, and in several of the cases two, and even three, operations have had to be performed before the opening could be closed.

To get over these objections, and still give rest to the colon, ileo-sigmoidostomy has been performed with the object of short-circuiting the colon. This has been done successfully in several cases. B. V. Beck has performed it for chronic colitis in six cases. The results were excellent in five, but in the sixth the patient died as the result of a Murphy's button having been used for the anastomosis. This operation is the same as that which Lane has performed for constipation, and it is possible that some of his cases were of the same nature.

Ileo-sigmoidostomy is much to be preferred to a right-sided colotomy, but is severe considering the nature of the malady, and has the further objection that it permanently short-circuits the colon, and the normal course for the fæces cannot afterwards be re-established. There is, however, considerable difference of opinion as to whether this is an objection or not. Also, in many cases the rectum and sigmoid flexure are involved in the disease, in fact are often the most diseased, and consequently the operation will not short-circuit the entire diseased area. Ileo-sigmoidostomy is, moreover, for other reasons an unsatisfactory operation, but this will be discussed in considering that operation.

Left inguinal colotomy has also been done; but this operation has nothing to recommend it, as it does not get above the disease and cannot, therefore, do much good. The objections to a right-sided artificial anus in these cases were early recognized, and the plan of making a valvular opening into the cæcum, through which the fæces would not escape, but through which the colon could be effectually washed out, was tried. Gibson was one of the first to perform this operation, and it proved quite satisfactory as regards a cure of the colitis. Except in exceptional cases, however, it has been replaced by the operation of appendicostomy, by which the same object is more readily attained.

Appendicostomy has none of the objections of right-sided colotomy, and the results of this operation in the treatment of chronic colitis seem to be equally satisfactory.

The operation is practically free from risk, does not prevent the patient from attending to his ordinary occupation, and does not cause any discomfort or even inconvenience. It is therefore a suitable operation in these cases. I have collected several cases in which appendicostomy was performed for this condition.

Case.—A man, aged 35, was under my care in St. Mark's Hospital in 1907. For fifteen months he had been suffering from repeated severe attacks of pain in the abdomen, accompanied by the passage of much mucus. He had been unable to follow his occupation, and a long course of medical treatment had given him no material relief. Appendicostomy was performed and the colon washed out daily with two pints of boracic lotion, and later with the same quantity of water. Previous to operation, the colon could be seen on examination with the sigmoidoscope to be much inflamed, and in several places ulcers were present. After the operation his symptoms quickly cleared up, and a month later all signs of inflammation in the colon had disappeared. He left the hospital and continued the irrigations for six months; meanwhile, however, he returned to his occupation. Three months after operation he had gained over a stone in weight and felt quite well. A year after the operation he was still quite well, and had had no return of the colitis. The opening of the appendix caused him no trouble, and he was advised to keep it open for some months longer. When last seen a few months ago he was quite well, and the opening had been allowed to close.

Case.—A lady, aged 32, had for eight years been a complete invalid owing to severe intermittent attacks of so-called membranous colitis. She spent most of her time in bed, was highly neurotic, and had lost weight. She had been treated by different dietaries, and douches, medicine, and electricity, but without any improvement. Sigmoidoscopy showed chronic inflammation of the mucous membrane.

I performed exploratory laparotomy, which revealed some thickening of the bowel wall and adhesions binding down the sigmoid flexure. The latter were divided and appendicostomy performed. The colon was daily irrigated with water, and the patient continued the irrigation for herself after her return home. She rapidly improved and put on weight. Six months later she was quite well, and there had been no further attacks of colitis and no mucus or membrane in the stools. I heard from her again over a year after the operation; she was quite well and had had no return of the colitis.

This case is of particular interest, as the patient previous to operation was very bad, and the question of making an artificial anus on the right side had been discussed. A complete cure of the condition resulted from the operation, and has remained permanent up to the present time.

I have collected in all twenty cases in which appendicostomy was performed for chronic colitis. These include six cases of my own, of which five were operated upon by myself, and one by another surgeon before I saw the case. There are also fourteen cases collected from medical records. The results in these cases may be tabulated, as follows:—

Cases.		Results.		Remarks.
Author	6	Cured	4	All well over a year later. There were slight temporary relapses in two cases.
		Improved	1	
		No better	1	
Edwards	1	Cured		
Tuttle	2	Cured	1	
		Improved	1	
Willis	1	Cured		
Keetley	3	Cured	2	
Moynihan	1	Cured		
Armour	1	Cured		
Stretton	3	Cured	1	
		Improved	1	
		No better	1	
Grey	1	Recovered		Slight relapse two years later.
Pringle	1	No better		

In 13 out of the 20 cases the patients were cured of the colitis, and no relapse is stated to have occurred. In three the patients much improved, but one or more slight and temporary relapses occurred during the following two years. In three the patients were no better after the operation; and one was too recent to form any opinion.

The three cases in which there was no improvement are worth recording in detail. The first was a lady, aged 32, who was sent to me by her medical attendant with a history that appendicostomy had been performed for chronic colitis a year previously, but that she had not been any better since the operation. A careful examination of the bowel with the sigmoidoscope showed no signs of colitis, and I came to the conclusion that she had some lesion in the hepatic flexure of the colon, probably adhesions from an old gastric ulcer. She was averse to any further operation.

The second is a case, reported by Mr. Seton Pringle,* of a labouring man with severe membranous colitis, on whom appendicostomy was performed. No improvement followed the operation, and six months later he was as bad as before. An examination of the bowel with the sigmoidoscope showed no colitis.

Mr. Stretton reported the third case. The patient was an elderly woman, on whom appendicostomy was performed for symptoms which were attributed to chronic mucous colitis. No improvement followed the operation, and it was subsequently discovered that there was a malignant growth in the sigmoid flexure which had been the cause of the symptoms. It thus seems probable that the cases where no improvement follows appendicostomy are those in which a wrong diagnosis has been made in the first instance. In some of the cases in which relapse has occurred, this has apparently been due to the opening being closed too soon.

From these instances, few as they are, it may, I think, be fairly concluded that in appendicostomy we possess a very good and useful means of treating bad cases of true chronic colitis which will not respond satisfactorily to medical treatment ; by it we may expect to obtain a cure of the condition without serious risk, and without inconvenience, even in the worst and most protracted cases.

I purposely say true chronic colitis, for if the operation is performed without a correct diagnosis having previously been made, and therefore on patients in whom the symptoms are due to some gross lesion of the colon, a satisfactory result cannot be expected. Where there is chronic inflammation of the colon, a good result may confidently be expected from the operation, and where chronic colitis is associated with, or has resulted from, a gross lesion, good results will follow, providing the lesion is removed or remedied at the same time.

---

* *Brit. Med. Jour.* 1908, vol. ii, p. 1713.

It is certainly advisable that the opening should not be closed too hastily, and a year, or even longer, is not too much to allow before permanently closing the appendix. The disease is one which is particularly liable to relapse, even after long periods of complete immunity from all symptoms; and as the operation cannot readily be repeated, it is advisable to retain the opening until all likelihood of a relapse has passed.

If in nine months after the operation there has been no recurrence of symptoms, the irrigations may be discontinued, and the opening allowed to close of itself. This it will do in a few days by the formation of a thin skin over the externa opening. In this condition it will not cause the slightest inconvenience, and if later there should arise the necessity to re-open it, this can readily be done by the introduction of a probe, because the appendix itself will not have closed.

Many people seem to have an idea that appendicostomy results in an objectionable condition somewhat like that following colotomy. This is, however, not the case. If the operation has been properly performed, there is nothing but a small and depressed scar in the abdominal wall, from which neither fæces nor mucus escapes, and over which in most cases it is not necessary to wear anything except the ordinary underclothing. The patient should be quite unaware of the presence of any opening except when using it for irrigation, and it does not prevent the patient living an ordinary life. For details of the operation the reader is referred to the chapter on appendicostomy.

All kinds of fluids have been used for the purpose of irrigating the colon, and in three cases which have come under my observation, symptoms of poisoning have resulted. Two were cases of boracic acid poisoning, and one of carboluria from the use of lysol. Antiseptics do not seem to be necessary, and some of the best results have been attained where nothing but plain water was used; when patients have to do the irrigation for themselves, this is much to be preferred. Silver compounds, such as argyrol or protargol, 0·5 or 1 per cent, have been employed, but are probably unnecessary.

In conclusion, it may be said that the first essential for successful treatment is a correct diagnosis: this necessitates an examination with the sigmoidoscope, and sometimes may require an exploratory laparotomy. In true chronic colitis appendicostomy should be the operation of choice in all cases where medical treatment has failed.

ENTEROSPASM.

This is the name given to a condition in which there is a spasmodic contraction of the circular muscle-fibres in some portion of the colon. The contraction of the colon is localized to one spot, and varies from one to several inches in length. So intense is the constriction, that the bowel lumen is partly or completely closed, and symptoms of intestinal obstruction occur. The condition is comparable to asthma and spasmodic stricture of the urethra.

It is only recently that anything positive has been known about this curious condition, but before it was described, many surgeons had met with cases in which a patient with all the symptoms of intestinal obstruction had been operated upon, and on opening the abdomen no obstruction of any sort was discovered after the most careful search. In several of such cases the upper part of the colon and small bowel were found distended, and the lower portion of the colon collapsed and empty; yet no obstruction or possible cause of obstruction was to be discovered at the point where the distended and collapsed bowel joined. These cases were a mystery, but it now seems probable that they were in reality instances of enterospasm. Although enterospasm was first suggested as an explanation of these and similar cases on purely negative evidence, we now have positive proof that the condition actually occurs.

In not a few cases the spasmodic stricture has been seen and handled during an operation for the relief of intestinal obstruction. Perhaps the best instance occurred in the practice of my colleague, Mr. Swinford Edwards. The patient was a woman with a history of several attacks of partial obstruction in the colon. Careful palpation of the abdomen revealed the presence of a hard swelling apparently in the sigmoid flexure, and it was thought that she had a tumour obstructing this portion of the colon. It was decided to perform laparotomy, and, if possible, remove the growth. On opening the abdomen, Mr. Edwards was unable to find any tumour, and the sigmoid flexure appeared to be normal. While, however, he was examining it, a contraction about two inches in length appeared in the sigmoid flexure.

The contracted portion was hard, and might easily have given the impression of a tumour when felt through the abdominal wall. The contraction disappeared and then re-appeared in the same place while the colon was under observation.

I have also had a similar case in my own practice. The patient was a woman, aged 39, who was admitted into the hospital for attacks of intense abdominal pain and symptoms of a severe colitis. A sausage-shaped tumour about two inches long could be felt in the region of the sigmoid flexure. There was constant diarrhœa, with stools consisting of blood and mucus. I at first thought there was a growth in the bowel which had caused the symptoms, but a careful examination revealed the fact that the tumour was only present during attacks of abdominal pain, and that when the patient was examined between the attacks no tumour could be felt. This was verified by repeated examinations, and we came to the conclusion that the supposed tumour was due to a localized contraction of the colon. The affected portion of colon always occupied the same position, and was appearently of the same size. There was tenderness on pressure over this spot, and in view of this, and the presence of blood in the stools, it seemed probable that the enterospasm was set up by an ulcer in the colon. The patient was treated by dietary and full doses of belladonna. She recovered, and left the hospital free from the attacks of pain from which she had previously suffered.

Etiology.

The patients are nearly always women between the ages of thirty and fifty, and usually of a markedly neurotic type. There is a history of hysteria, or other symptoms ascribed to neurasthenia, in almost all cases. The condition is closely associated with chronic colitis, and I have never met with a case in which there were not well-marked symptoms of colitis.

There is good reason to suppose that the spasm is set up by some local lesion in the colon. Thus the condition is always accompanied by a chronic colitis. Moreover, in all the cases which I have seen or been able to find recorded, there has been blood in the stools, which is definite evidence of ulceration somewhere in the bowel. The fact that the spasm is localized to a particular portion of the bowel also strongly suggests a local irritative cause.

The condition is essentially a chronic one, and there is usually a history of attacks of abdominal pain dating back for several years.

Symptoms.

The most marked symptom is severe abdominal pain. This usually occurs in paroxysms, which commence suddenly without apparent cause, and after lasting for a period varying from a few hours to several days, pass off equally suddenly. The pain while it lasts is very severe, and often closely resembles that which occurs in the early stages of peritonitis or acute intestinal obstruction. It may also be easily mistaken for renal colic. It is usually well localized to that portion of the abdomen in which the contracted area of colon lies. Vomiting not infrequently accompanies the pain, and may be well marked. If the spasm continues for any length of time, the abdomen becomes distended, there is more or less complete constipation, and the patient's condition becomes typical of acute intestinal obstruction. Either as the result of the administration of morphia, or naturally, the attack suddenly terminates, the bowels act, the pain stops, and in a few hours the patient is quite well again. If the abdomen is examined during an attack, it is often possible to feel the contracted area of colon, which is most commonly situated in the descending colon or sigmoid flexure.

In addition to the symptoms caused by the enterospasm, there are usually those of a chronic colitis. The stools contain much mucus and often blood. There is constipation alternating with periods of diarrhœa, and all the other symptoms usually associated with a chronic colitis. In the more severe cases fæcal vomiting and visible peristalsis may also be present.

The diagnosis is extremely difficult. The condition may be suspected, but if the patient is first seen during an attack it will be practically impossible to be certain that the condition is due to enterospasm. The greatest difficulty arises in deciding as to whether or not an operation shall be performed. Usually the condition, though very distressing, is not serious, but the following case, reported by Dr. Pendred,[*] terminated fatally.

Case.—The patient was a querulous, excitable woman, aged 57. For the preceding three years she had suffered from time to time

---

Brit. Med. Jour., May 29, 1909, p. 1292.

ENTEROSPASM

from colic, with vomiting and diarrhœa. Latterly these attacks had become very frequent and severe. The urine showed a trace of albumin, and she complained of frequent micturition. During the next two months, in spite of energetic treatment, she had much colic, and had plainly emaciated. A copious bleeding from the rectum occurred about this time. Month after month she continued to waste, and had constant vomiting attacks. Constipation alternated with diarrhœa, which latter somewhat relieved her pain.

In July, 1905—ten months after she was first seen—she was nearly bedridden with colic, coming on every few minutes, accompanied by tremendous borborygmi. Visible peristaltic waves passed across coils of intestine from left to right every few minutes, as though the intestine were endeavouring to overcome some obstruction. By the end of this month her condition was pitiable, and she had to be kept constantly under the influence of morphine. The pain was almost constant night and day. The vomit now became stercoraceous, hiccough supervened, and the bowels were confined. On July 29th the abdomen was opened, but at first nothing amiss could be found. At one point the distention of the gut suddenly ceased, and the distal portion was flat, toneless, and of a paler colour, so that it was thought the obstruction had been discovered. Whilst the bowel was being watched, the collapsed gut began to fill out again, just as it had appeared to do through the abdominal wall. Three days later her condition was as bad as ever, the gurgling, peristalsis, pain, and sickness, with occasional hæmatemesis, being nearly continuous. She died in the middle of September. A post-mortem examination of the abdomen showed that every organ, though wasted, was macroscopically healthy. The intestine was partly opened up, and presented a normal appearance.

TREATMENT.

The obvious treatment, if the condition can be diagnosed, is to give a full dose of morphia and belladonna to allay the spasm. This will usually quickly terminate the attack. Placing the patient in a hot bath will also often have a similar effect. But the key to the situation is the diagnosis, and it is often impossible to be certain that we are not dealing with a strangulation of the bowel.

If the condition can be diagnosed, further attacks may be prevented by treating the colitis and by administering belladonna in full doses.

Chapter XII.

ULCERATIVE COLITIS.

UNTIL quite recently ulcerative colitis was a disease of the post-mortem table; it was seldom diagnosed during life (with the exception of tropical dysentery), and no attempt had been made to deal with it by operative surgery. It is now, however, beginning to be recognized that ulceration of the colon may be dealt with successfully, and already there are a number of cases on record in which the disease has been cured by operation, which otherwise would almost certainly have ended fatally.

The subject of ulcerative colitis is surrounded by many difficulties. Most of our knowledge of the morbid appearances is derived from post-mortem examinations, in which from the nature of things only the terminal and most severe characters of the disease can be studied. The confusion which exists between ulcerative colitis and tropical dysentery is as yet far from being cleared up, and there are those who still assert that all cases of ulcerative colitis are examples of tropical dysentery.

Ulceration of the colon resembles that of the skin, inasmuch as it may result from a great many different conditions and occur in many different forms. Thus it may arise secondarily to some constitutional trouble, such as Bright's disease, gout or plumbism. It may result from a specific infection, as in amœbic dysentery, Shiga's bacillary dysentery, enteric fever, tuberculosis, and possibly syphilis. It may occur from malignant disease, or as the result of hardened and long-retained fæcal masses, such as the ulceration caused by a stercolith, or in the dilated bowel above a stricture. It may follow damage to the blood-supply of the colon, as in some cases of cirrhosis of the liver and in embolism of the mesenteric arteries. Or it may result from trophic changes due to interference with the innervation of the colon; two such cases are

ULCERATIVE COLITIS

recorded by Dr. Hale White, in which the patient had a fractured spine and paraplegia.

Much of the confusion which surrounds the subject has arisen from the fact that investigators have often failed to sufficiently recognize the great number of different causes of ulceration in the colon, and, confusing several together, have attributed all to some specific cause.

Ulcerative colitis has been considered so fatal a disease, apart from tropical dysentery, that some writers have maintained it cannot be recovered from, and that the reported cases of recovery were not true ulcerative colitis. This is a not uncommon error when a disease is studied only upon the post-mortem table and there is no other means of arriving at a correct diagnosis. A study of the recorded cases would

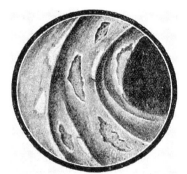

Fig. 44.—Ulcers in the sigmoid flexure in a case of chronic constipation.

certainly lead to the conclusion that the disease, except in its epidemic form, is practically always fatal.

The sigmoidoscope, however, has made it possible to diagnose ulcerative colitis with certainty without a post-mortem examination, and it is now obvious that the disease is by no means incompatible with complete recovery, and with early diagnosis and suitable operative interference there is good reason to hope that much may be done to materially lower the mortality.

ETIOLOGY.

The disease is one of early adult life; thus, out of my series of 60 cases, the average age is 37. It apparently does not occur in children, with the exception of follicular colitis.

The sexes appear to be equally affected; out of the total of 177 cases collected from different London hospitals at the time of the discussion on ulcerative colitis, which took place in January, 1909, at the Royal Society of Medicine, 89 were males and 88 females.

BACTERIOLOGY.

Ulcerative colitis necessarily includes endemic amœbic dysentery and epidemic bacillary dysentery, or, as it is sometimes called, asylum dysentery.

The former is a well-marked and distinct endemic form of ulcerative colitis which does not occur in this country, and for further information in reference to it the reader is referred to works on tropical medicine.

A great deal of work has recently been done upon the subject of bacillary dysentery, and the organisms which are supposed to cause the disease have been separated. The most important of these are Shiga's *Bacillus dysenteriæ*, and Flexner's acid bacillus. They have not, however, fulfilled Koch's postulates, and there is not at present sufficient proof to establish the specific bacteriological origin of ulcerative colitis. Many investigators have maintained that chronic ulcerative colitis and bacillary dysentery are the same disease; some have even gone so far as to maintain that the cases of chronic ulcerative colitis met with in this country are sporadic cases of amœbic dysentery; but the latter is certainly not true, except, perhaps, in a few isolated instances, as the amœbæ cannot be demonstrated in the stools, nor do the cases bear any but a superficial clinical resemblance to cases of dysentery.

Supporting the view of a close relationship between bacillary dysentery and chronic ulcerative colitis, Dr. Carver has pointed out that, both at the Great Northern Hospital in 1902, and at the Westminster Hospital in 1903, an outbreak of acute bacillary dysentery followed the admission into these hospitals of cases of chronic ulcerative colitis. As yet, however, it has certainly not been proved that ulcerative colitis is due to a specific bacterial infection, and it is at present impossible to say whether the organisms discovered in the ulcers are the cause of the ulceration or are a secondary infection. Flexner and Sweet have shown that in cases of bacillary dysentery the lesions in the colon are apparently produced by the elimination of toxins.

PLATE IV

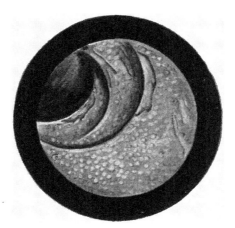

Fig. A.—CHRONIC ULCERATIVE COLITIS, with much thickening of the bowel-wall and a granular condition of the mucosa, as seen through the sigmoidoscope.

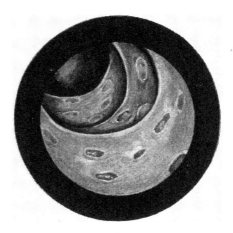

Fig. B.

Fig. B.—Appearances in a case of FOLLICULAR COLITIS.

ULCERATIVE COLITIS

The toxins are excreted chiefly by the large intestine, and it is the reaction to this process which produces the lesions.

PATHOLOGY.

Many different types of ulceration are seen in the colon, and it is not at present possible to say whether they are different kinds of ulceration, or only different degrees of the same type.

In some cases the mucous membrane is so destroyed by ulceration that little normal membrane can be seen anywhere in the entire colon, while in others there are only a few isolated ulcers in one or more parts of it. In the majority of cases in which a post-mortem examination has been made, the entire colon was more or less ulcerated. In most of the records I have been able to find, the colon was the only part diseased,

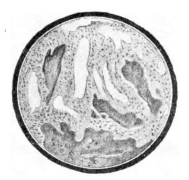

Fig. 45.—Ulcerative colitis—sigmoidoscopic

except for septic lesions such as abscess, or peritonitis, the secondary consequence of the ulceration.

The lesions vary in size, from quite small, punched-out ulcers, the size of a pea, up to large irregular tracts covering many inches. When examined during life with the sigmoidoscope, the edges of the ulcers can be seen to be raised, and to have a bright red areola. The base is generally covered with fine granulations, and there is often either white adherent mucus or a yellow slough adhering to the surface. These sloughs, however, quickly become detached by the constant diarrhœa, and consequently are not commonly found in post-mortem specimens.

The ulcers are most often seen, and appear to commence, in the hollows of the bowel, such as in the depressions between the valvulæ conniventes, and in the bases of the sacculi. When the disease is extensive, the ulcers tend to run together, and become confluent, so that they assume a most irregular outline. Small islands of normal mucosa often remain in places, and stand out like polypi above the surrounding ulceration; similarly, narrow bands or bridges of mucous membrane may be left between the ulcers, and this often gives the bowel a most curious appearance. At first sight it appears as though covered with polypi, but a closer inspection shows these to consist of islands of swollen mucous membrane surrounded by ulceration. In some cases the ulceration has spread almost uniformly over the bowel, in others longitudinally, leaving long ridges of normal mucosa standing above the surrounding ulcerated surface. Again, the ulceration may have spread circularly.

Occasionally the ulcers are all more or less discrete, though numerous, and the appearance is as if the mucosa was honeycombed or trabeculated. They are commonly numerous, and extend throughout the greater part, if not the whole, of the colon; but in a few cases there have been not more than one or two large ulcers.

The depth of the lesions varies considerably: in some the mucosa appears as if scraped or sandpapered, so that the surface is entirely removed. This condition is seen in cases examined with the sigmoidoscope, and probably represents an earlier or milder stage of the disease than is observed in the postmortem specimens. The surface is raw, bleeding, and has a granular appearance (see *Plate IV, Fig. A*). Often the greater part of the mucosa is destroyed; in severe cases the muscular coat is exposed in the base of the ulcers, while in some the floor of the ulcer is formed by peritoneum only. In the chronic type there is usually considerable thickening of the bowel-wall from fibrous tissue.

If the ulcers have perforated the muscular coat, there may be some local peritonitis and adherent lymph on the outside of the bowel. The mesenteric glands may be enlarged, and this was noted in several of the recorded cases, though in many there was no glandular enlargement.

There is nothing distinctive in the microscopical appearances of ulcerative colitis. Sections of the wall of the colon through

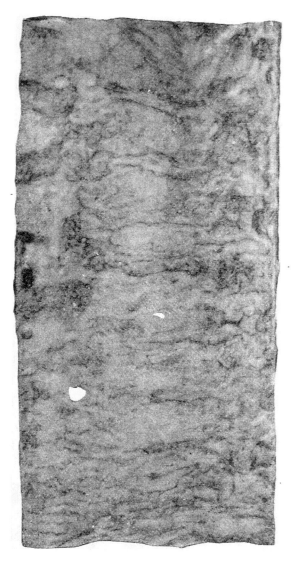

Fig. 46.—Ulcerative colitis, showing the mucous membrane entirely destroyed down to the muscular coat, except for a few isolated islands here and there. (*From a specimen in Charing Cross Hospital Museum.*)

an ulcerated area show the ordinary characters of simple inflammation. In the less severe cases the glands of Lieberkühn are seen to have undergone cloudy swelling and to contain fibrinous material in their lumen. The submucosa is usually much thickened, highly vascular, and there is a general round-celled infiltration. The muscular coat is infiltrated with leucocytes, and where the ulceration is deep the fibres are destroyed. The peritoneum is thickened.

Where the ulceration has extended through the whole depth of the mucosa, the islets of mucous membrane left between the ulcers can be seen to have become thickened and swollen, with the result that, under the microscope, they present the appearance of polypi covered with mucous membrane. In some instances the ulceration can be seen to have extended under the mucous membrane, leaving it attached by a narrow stalk.

The causes of death in the cases which I have been able to collect were as follows :—

	CASES.
Perforation and general peritonitis	9
Exhaustion	17
Pyæmia	4
Embolism	2
Anuria	1

Perforation is thus a common cause of death. In nearly all, the ulcer which had perforated was in the cæcum or sigmoid flexure; in only one was there a perforation in the transverse colon, and in that a large portion of the transverse colon had sloughed right away. In two cases there was more than one perforation. In one a perforation into the general peritoneal cavity was present in both the cæcum and sigmoid flexure, and in the other there was an ulcer in the cæcum the size of a shilling opening straight into the peritoneal cavity, and five or six others, also perforating, in the cæcum and ascending colon. It is difficult to see how more than one perforation can occur, but it is possible that some sudden strain or distention of the bowel with gas caused several ulcers to give way at the same time.

Perforation of an ulcer may occur without causing general peritonitis; in several of the cases a local abscess or pericolitis had resulted, and was shut off by adhesions from the general peritoneal cavity. In one there was a large abscess in the pelvis communicating by several large perforations with the interior of the cæcum. In another there was a pericolic abscess in connection with the sigmoid flexure due to an ulcer which had perforated. In one case the bases of some of the ulcers had become adherent to neighbouring coils of small bowel, and perforation had occurred into the small bowel. There was a communication between the ascending colon and the small intestine, and another between the ascending colon and the ileum.

Adhesions between different coils of bowel or between the colon and the parietal peritoneum are not uncommon, and once or twice it was found post mortem, on separating the adhesions, that several ulcers had perforated.

Although abscess of the liver is a common complication of amœbic dysentery, it is uncommon in other forms of ulcerative colitis, and was only present in two of the cases I have collected. In one of these the abscess was single, in the other there were multiple abscesses. Neither of these patients had ever been out of England, and there was no reason to suppose they had amœbic dysentery. One would expect portal pyæmia to be a common complication, but out of nearly sixty cases it was present in these two only. In one other instance there were symptoms of liver abscess, but the patient recovered without operation.

Hæmorrhage serious enough to threaten life may result from an ulcer opening up an artery, and in hæmorrhagic colitis the bleeding is the most serious symptom. General peritonitis may result from ulcerative colitis without any perforation being present.

SYMPTOMS.

The main symptom in all cases is diarrhœa; and it is this which draws attention to the disease. It may begin suddenly, accompanied by severe abdominal pain, or, rarely, may come on insidiously with a slight looseness of the bowels. Usually the patient states that the pain and diarrhœa started quite suddenly, without any very apparent cause. The stools increase in frequency, and blood appears. The ordinary remedies as a rule have no affect upon the diarrhœa, and the patient rapidly loses weight and becomes extremely ill. The number of stools varies considerably. A common number is six to eight, and I have seen several instances where there were twenty, in the twenty-four hours. The stools are quite watery, and contain comparatively little fæcal material, consisting mostly of mucus, blood, pus, water, and undigested food. In a severe case of ulcerative colitis the food passes through the alimentary tract with surprising rapidity. If charcoal is given with the food, we can easily ascertain how long any particular feed has taken in traversing the alimentary canal, as the excreta will be coloured black. If this test is applied, it will be found that a feed will sometimes appear in the stools in as short a time as three hours. It is not surprising, therefore, that in bad cases we sometimes see milk in the stools almost in the condition in which it was swallowed. In the worst cases the patient is practically unable to digest anything, and wasting and loss of weight are in consequence rapid and severe.

The amount of blood in the stools varies; in some cases it is considerable, while in others it is only present occasionally in small quantities. It is usually fluid, and intimately mixed with the stool: it may, however, appear as small, jelly-like clots.

The desire to go to stool is sudden and urgent, but defæcation is not as a rule accompanied by tenesmus. Personally I have never seen a patient with ulcerative colitis in whom there was well-marked tenesmus, and although some writers give it as a common symptom, I believe it to be exceptional. When present, it points to severe ulceration in the rectum. In acute tropical dysentery, however, tenesmus is a common symptom.

There is not infrequently considerable abdominal pain and tenderness. The pain is referred to the abdominal wall, but is not well localized. The tenderness is most marked in the left iliac fossa and in the left loin, but often extends over the whole colon.

The character of the stools varies considerably, but they are always thin, watery, and contain blood. Pus is seldom present in any large amount, but can always be detected on microscopical examination. There is always mucus, and often sloughs can be seen if the stools are carefully examined. They are usually very fœtid. The digestion is much disturbed, and nausea and vomiting may occur and cause considerable distress. Vomiting is, however, exceptional, except in the more acute cases, and, indeed, many patients suffering from chronic ulcerative colitis have surprisingly few symptoms apart from the diarrhœa and consequent loss of weight. I have even seen patients with the pelvic colon, showing extensive and severe ulceration, who were able to get about and who complained only of the constant diarrhœa.

The progress of the disease varies a good deal. Some patients get rapidly worse, go steadily downhill from the first, lose much weight, seem unable to digest anything, and in a few weeks become wasted skeletons. Others seem to go on for months, sometimes a little better, and sometimes worse. Others again, after a severe attack lasting several weeks or months, get better and remain well for a time, only to have renewed attacks which, as a rule, are more severe.

The condition usually described is that in which the symptoms soon become serious, and the patient's life is threatened; but it is important to recognize that there are other types of chronic ulcerative colitis in which the symptoms are never very severe, and the patient is able to get about, though frequently troubled with diarrhœa. It has been stated that where the symptoms are comparatively mild the condition is not ulcerative colitis; but frequent examinations with the sigmoidoscope have convinced me that very extensive ulceration may and often does exist, though it seems probable that the ulceration is confined to the pelvic colon.

The temperature is commonly, though not invariably, raised. Except in the more severe cases it is not high, but varies between 100° F. and 101° F. The chart, if examined, usually shows a very irregular temperature of the type we generally associate with chronic septic poisoning. I have seen several cases, however, in which, although there was severe diarrhœa and the sigmoidoscope showed extensive ulceration, the temperature never rose over 99° F. while the patient was under observation. These were, however, all very chronic cases, in which the symptoms had existed for months or years. All observers agree that relapses are very common in those cases which are not fatal. When death occurs it is usually due to exhaustion and wasting; less frequently to perforation and general peritonitis; and in a few instances to hæmorrhage. At the present day the diagnosis should not be difficult, as the pelvic colon is always involved, and this can be directly examined with the sigmoidoscope. The instrument must, however, be used with great care, because the bowel wall is weak and friable. In experienced hands there is no risk in using the sigmoidoscope; but no one who is unaccustomed to the instrument should attempt an examination in suspected ulcerative colitis. (*Plate IV, Fig. A.*)

The disease can, as a rule, be diagnosed from the symptoms; but unless the sigmoidoscope is employed there are several conditions with which it can easily be confused. The most important of these is cancer of the pelvic colon or upper end of the rectum, which not infrequently gives rise to identical symptoms. Another is a high-lying fibrous stricture with secondary ulceration in the bowel above. The condition may also be confused with enteric fever, and with acute proctitis.

Acute tropical amœbic dysentery is not met with in this country, and its symptoms and treatment are so well described in modern works on tropical medicine, that it will not be discussed here. Cases of chronic dysentery are, however, not infrequently seen; but they differ in no important particular, either as regards symptoms or treatment, from chronic ulcerative colitis, except that when amœbæ can be demonstrated in the stools improvement often follows a course of special treatment by ipecacuanha.

NATURAL HEALING OF ULCERS IN THE COLON.—It is difficult to find any signs of repair in the specimens of ulcerative colitis beyond some thickening of the bowel-wall and a little adherent lymph on the peritoneum. Occasionally pigmented spots are seen in the colon which have been supposed to be the remains of old ulcers. One would expect that when an ulcer of the colon of any size healed, a considerable scar would be left and there would be a tendency to contraction and stricture. This appears, however, to be very rare. In the formation of scars the mucous lining of the bowel appears to behave very differently from the skin. We know that quite large ulcers in the small intestine due to enteric fever will heal and leave practically no scar, and certainly no stricture or contraction of the bowel-wall. And it is a very striking fact that if the interior of the bowel is examined some year or more after an operation, such, for instance, as an anastomosis, has been performed, the scar is often almost undetectable. I have on several occasions examined the interior of the sigmoid flexure with the sigmoidoscope after a portion has been resected, and been almost unable to find the line of union, so slight was the scar.

In a number of cases of ulceration of the colon I have been able with the sigmoidoscope to watch from time to time the process of repair in ulcers which could be seen in the sigmoid flexure. These ulcers can be seen gradually to diminish in size until only a slight white mark is left, and if examined a little later, even this has disappeared, leaving no perceptible scar. I have seen ulcers as large as a sixpence which looked quite deep, and which apparently exposed or even involved the muscular coat, disappear without leaving any obvious scar. Apparently it is only when the ulceration is very deep, involving the muscular coat, and also very extensive, that any appreciable scar results.

I have only twice been able with certainty to trace a stricture of the colon to a previous ulceration. But though this is very uncommon, there are several specimens in museums of fibrous stricture in the colon, in which it seems almost certain that the stricture is due to ulcerative colitis. It is not uncommon to see a tight fibrous stricture occur in the rectum as the result of extensive ulceration, and the same thing doubtless occasionally occurs in the colon. It seems probable that most cases of ulcerative colitis in which the ulceration is sufficiently severe to cause contraction, die from the initial disease. On one occasion I examined with the sigmoidoscope a woman who gave a history of previous bowel trouble which suggested ulceration in the pelvic colon, and I was able to see a narrow ring stricture in the middle of the sigmoid flexure, evidently of a fibrous nature, and which appeared probably to have resulted from the contraction of a healed ulcer. A case is reported by Dr. Tooth, of a woman who died from chronic ulcerative colitis in St. Bartholomew's Hospital; the colon was extensively ulcerated, and there was a contraction of the bowel at the splenic flexure.

Quénu records a death from intestinal obstruction due to a simple ulcer at the lower end of the sigmoid, which had contracted and caused a stricture.

Prognosis.

The prognosis is distinctly bad unless an operation is performed. A majority of the cases die, and the mortality is very high. The more extensive use of the sigmoidoscope, however, has proved that many recover, and that the condition is not so fatal as was previously supposed when a post-mortem examination was the only certain means of diagnosis.

With non-operative treatment, recovery, even if it occurs, is very slow, and recurrence in a few months extremely common. In the more acute cases, the prognosis is so grave that no time should be wasted in a preliminary trial of non-operative measures, but operation should be performed at once before the patient has become seriously weakened by the disease. Out of 80 cases which were admitted to St. Thomas's Hospital between the years 1883 and 1907, 50 per cent died, and the condition of the remainder was as follows :—

  No improvement 14
  Improved, but symptoms persisting 19
  Cure or great improvement 7

Thus only 7 cases out of 80 showed any marked improvement as the result of treatment, and of these 7, 5 were apparently treated by operation.

  Follicular Ulceration.—This is generally considered a distinct form of ulcerative colitis. The ulcers are small and discrete. They start by swelling and inflammation of the solitary follicles of the mucosa; the central portion then sloughs and leaves a small crater-like ulcer with a bright red areola. The ulcers do not extend deeply; they are circular in outline, with well-marked edges. They are always multiple. They may enlarge to about the size of a pea, but are seldom larger than this, and are never confluent; but it is by no means certain that the more extensive ulcers do not sometimes originate in follicular ulceration. I have not found any case in which this form of ulceration has caused perforation. (See *Plate IV, Fig. B.*)

  This form of ulcerative colitis occurs as a complication of other diseases. It is chiefly of interest here because it occurs in association with cancer of the alimentary canal. I have found it so associated in three cases. In one there was cancer of the stomach and follicular ulceration of the whole colon. In one there were numerous follicular ulcers *below* a cancerous stricture of the sigmoid; and in the third case there was epithelioma of the anus.

  SYMPTOMS AND PROGNOSIS.—The symptoms are the same as in other forms of chronic ulcerative colitis, but are much less severe when the condition occurs in adults. It is a not uncommon form of acute colitis in children, and many of the summer

ULCERATIVE COLITIS

diarrhœas which yearly account for so much of the infant mortality in the east end of London are of this nature.

Hæmorrhagic Colitis.—I have included this condition in the chapter on ulcerative colitis because it most conveniently comes under that heading, though strictly speaking there is not always any definite ulceration. It is a very rare form of colitis, and at present very little is known about it. It is an extremely serious and often fatal disease, and there are not sufficient cases at present available to enable us to draw any reliable conclusions as to its etiology. It appears to be a form of so-called bacillary dysentery, as everything points to a microbic infection as the cause. It occurs in young adults, and arises suddenly without any apparent cause. The characteristic symptoms are profuse and continuous hæmorrhage from the bowel, and uncontrollable diarrhœa. It closely resembles ulcerative colitis, and, like that disease, often starts suddenly with abdominal pain. There is profuse diarrhœa, and I have seen cases in which there were as many as twenty-five stools in the twenty-four hours. The amount of blood lost in the twenty-four hours may be very considerable, with the result that the patient rapidly becomes dangerously anæmic. All food passes almost straight through the intestine without being digested, and in a very short time the patient is reduced to an extreme condition of emaciation. The pulse is rapid and almost imperceptible, the temperature is raised, and the condition of the patient resembles that seen in a severe attack of typhoid fever during the third week of that illness. In one of my cases there was hyperpyrexia, the temperature going up to 109° F. on one occasion. The stools are liquid and extremely foul smelling. The blood is intimately mixed with them, and is present in such quantities that they are bright red in colour, often appearing to consist of little else but blood.

DIAGNOSIS AND SYMPTOMS.—The diagnosis can only be made with certainty by means of the sigmoidoscope. The appearance of the mucous membrane is characteristic, the whole surface being dark red and having a spongy appearance. Blood can be usually seen oozing from it everywhere. Definite ulcers may or may not be present, and this will depend to some extent on what is the stage of the disease at the time of examination.

The condition somewhat closely resembles enteric fever in symptomatology, and without a sigmoidoscopic examination might be mistaken for it. Widal's reaction is, however, not obtainable, and there are no spots; moreover, hæmorrhage is present from the beginning. I have no doubt, however, that many cases have been mistaken for typhoid fever.

The inflammation is not confined to the mucous membrane, but involves all the bowel-coats, and the peritoneum covering the bowel shows commencing peritonitis. The following is a good instance of this rare condition:—

The patient was a lady, aged 30. She was suddenly seized with severe abdominal pain, followed by diarrhœa. The stools contained blood and were very offensive. She continued to get about, but the diarrhœa increased, and at the end of a week she was having as many as fourteen stools daily, all of which contained blood. There was no further pain or other symptom except progressive weakness and emaciation. She came up to London and saw her doctor, who immediately sent her to bed and put her on a light diet. The bleeding, however, continued in spite of treatment, and she had a temperature ranging between 101° and 102°. I was asked to see her on the fifteenth day after the onset, and a sigmoidoscopic examination showed the mucosa of the pelvic colon to be spongy, bleeding, and of a dark-red colour. Hæmorrhagic colitis was diagnosed, and it was decided to perform appendicostomy in the hope of controlling the bleeding, which was already most serious. The operation was performed at once, and a large quantity of very foul material was washed out of the colon. The next day the patient's temperature, which had come down as the result of the operation, went up within an hour and a half to 109°, and was only got down again by continuous sponging and the application of ice, iced water being also run into the colon. For the next two days there were repeated attacks of hyperpyrexia, and on two occasions the temperature reached 107° before it could be checked. The bleeding from the colon was stopped in twenty-four hours as the result of frequent irrigation of the colon with water and 1 per cent argyrol. A specimen of the stools, which was examined bacteriologically, showed large numbers of pneumococci, which were also successfully cultivated, and the condition appeared to have been due to a primary infection of the colon by this organism. There were no symptoms of lung trouble. At the operation the cæcum, which was the only part of the large bowel examined, was found to be acutely inflamed, the wall was considerably thickened, and there was much adherent lymph on the peritoneal surface. As a result of frequent irrigation the colitis got better, and the stools became almost normal in appearance and free from blood. The temperature came down, and the patient seemed to be well on the way to recovery, when she died suddenly from heart failure.*

TREATMENT.—The best treatment in these cases, in fact the only treatment which seems to control the hæmorrhage, is to perform appendicostomy and keep the colon washed out. This rapidly controls the bleeding and at the same time washes away the highly toxic material in the colon, which, owing to the damaged condition of the bowel wall, is being absorbed and poisoning the patient. The condition is a very serious one, both on account of the great loss of blood and also the severe degree of toxæmia which results from it, and I am personally convinced that no time should be wasted in trying palliative measures, but appendicostomy should be performed as soon as possible after the condition has been diagnosed. The bowel should be washed out at once, and the washing continued until the fluid coming from the tube in the rectum is quite clean. After that, the colon should be irrigated every three or four hours until the hæmorrhage is controlled. Hazeline, in the proportion of two drachms to the pint, may be added to the water used for irrigation, and if this fails to stop the bleeding, the bowel may be washed through with 1 per cent argyrol.

During convalescence the feeding will require the most careful management, and, in fact, these cases call for every resource of modern medical knowledge and skill if they are to be conducted to a successful issue.

Distention or Stercoral Ulcers.—These are commonly found above a stricture of the colon or rectum. The most common situation is in the dilated portion of bowel immediately above the stricture; but they may occur in any part of the colon above the stricture; thus the stricture may be in the rectum, and the ulcer in the cæcum. They are usually multiple,

---

* *Proc. Roy. Soc. Med.*, vol. iii., No. 2, Clin. Sect., p. 48.

discrete ulcers with well-marked edges. They do not differ in any important particular as regards their morbid appearance from the form of ulceration already described. They apparently arise as the result of the local irritation and inflammation caused by retained fæcal material above the stricture. In fact, they may be said to be traumatic in origin. They are seen in cases of fæcal impaction when there is no stricture, and may occur as the result of chronic constipation alone. I have seen one such case in which several stercoral ulcers were present in the sigmoid flexure (see *Fig.* 44) of an old woman who for years had suffered from chronic constipation. They are for the most part quite shallow, and involve only the mucous membrane; but when they occur above a stricture they may in time expose the peritoneum, and perforate or give rise to local abscess formation.

Simple Perforating Ulcer of the Colon.—There are a few rare cases in which a patient has developed acute general peritonitis, and either at the time of operation or post mortem a single simple ulcer in the colon has been discovered which had perforated into the peritoneal cavity.

These cases do not appear to belong to the same class as those of ulcerative colitis which have previously been described, and I have therefore placed them separately, though it may subsequently transpire that they should not be so divided.

They bear a close resemblance to perforating duodenal and gastric ulcers. They are distinguished from ordinary ulcerative colitis in that there is only a single ulcer, or at most two, the remainder of the colon being healthy, and that there are none of the usual symptoms of ulcerative colitis; in fact, in many there do not appear to have been any definite symptoms until the sudden onset of general peritonitis.

In one case the patient, a man who was not known to have suffered from any bowel trouble, was operated upon for a stone in the bladder; he died three days after the operation, and post mortem there was found general peritonitis due to a simple ulcer in the splenic angle of the colon which had perforated.

In a case of Quénu's, the patient, who was suffering from acute pneumonia, developed acute abdominal pain on the fourteenth day of the illness, and died with symptoms of general peritonitis. Post mortem there was a single ulcer in the descending colon which had perforated, and also an ulcer in the stomach. In several there was a stricture or obstruction in the colon below the situation of the ulcer. In one, a volvulus of the sigmoid flexure had been operated upon and untwisted three days before an ulcer in the cæcum perforated.

In another case reported by Quénu, the patient died after an illness lasting seventeen days, with symptoms of perforation and peritonitis. Post mortem there was a single ulcer about one inch in diameter in the transverse colon, which had perforated ; there was also an ulcer in the stomach. In one case there was a simple ulcer the size of a shilling in the sigmoid flexure, which had perforated and caused an abscess ; the patient died from pyæmia.

I have been able to find records of eighteen such cases in which there was either a single ulcer in the colon, or two small ulcers close together, the remainder of the colon being quite free from ulceration. All but two were men, and their ages varied between 27 and 67.

The situation of the ulcer is shown in the following table :—

	Cases
Sigmoid flexure	7
Ascending colon or hepatic flexure	4
Descending colon or splenic flexure	5
Transverse colon	1
Cæcum	2

In three cases an obstruction existed below the ulcer. In one the ulcer was tuberculous, and one was due to typhoid fever. One patient was suffering from acute pneumonia ; but there is not positive evidence that the ulcer was caused by the pneumococcus. In the remaining cases there was present no apparent cause for the ulcer, and no other lesion of the colon. In most there was a history of constipation, but otherwise no trace of any bowel trouble until the sudden onset of symptoms of perforation. In one or two there was a history of localized pain and tenderness in the abdomen over the situation of the ulcer for a few weeks.

In one case two small concretions were found outside the bowel which had evidently come through the perforation. The ulcer had perforated the bowel wall in all but one of the cases, and had caused either an abscess or general peritonitis.

In a case reported by Dr. Bradbury, there was no apparent

perforation. The patient was a man, aged 30, who died after an illness which commenced with sudden pain in the abdomen. Post mortem there was a single small ulcer of the cæcum, which had not perforated. The appendix and the rest of the colon and small bowel were quite healthy. There were multiple abscesses of the liver and a right-sided empyema.

In two of the cases there was an ulcer in the stomach in addition to that in the colon. This is particularly interesting in view of the close resemblance which these ulcers of the colon bear to gastric ulcers. In three the lesion was undoubtedly a distention or stercoral ulcer occurring above a stricture or obstruction, and it seems possible that in many of the others the ulcer was of a traumatic nature, and caused by the retention for long periods of hardened fæcal masses.

In addition to the forms of perforating ulcer of the colon already mentioned, there are two others of importance. *Typhoid ulceration* of the colon is not common, but I have been able to collect seven cases in which a typhoid ulcer of the colon perforated and caused fatal peritonitis. In one case the ulcer was in the ascending colon, in two in the hepatic flexure, in two in the cæcum, and in two in the sigmoid flexure. *Tuberculous ulceration* of the colon may also result in perforation.

Treatment of Ulcerative Colitis.

Chronic ulcerative colitis is a disease about which, until quite recently, but little was known, and about which there is still much to learn. The cases have either had no special treatment or have been treated by restricted and special dietary, combined with attempts to wash out the lower bowel with antiseptic or silver solutions.

The cases treated by careful nursing and dietary, or by the administration of drugs, almost invariably died, and the only medical—as opposed to surgical—treatment which has been at all successful has been that in which an attempt has been made to wash out the bowel with weak solutions of antiseptics; though it cannot be said that even this has met with much success.

Dr. Hale White, in the discussion which took place at the Royal Society of Medicine on ulcerative colitis, stated that he knew of three cases which had apparently recovered as the result of treatment by coli vaccine.

Apparently the first instance of chronic ulcerative colitis

treated by operation was a case of Hahn's, in 1880. The patient was a prostitute, and it was at first supposed that the ulceration was due to syphilis, but as it did not improve under antisyphilitic treatment, he performed colotomy. Previous to operation she was very ill, and had lost 68 lbs. in weight, but she made a complete recovery. As the result of an attempt to close the artificial anus two years later, she died of pyæmia.

The first successful cæcostomy for ulcerative colitis seems to have been performed in Italy, in 1887, by Novara.

Of the 60 cases which I have been able to collect, 33 were treated medically and 27 by operation.

Of the cases not operated upon, 26 died and only seven recovered, while of those operated upon, 21 recovered, and only six died.

	Died.	Recovered.	Mortality per cent.
Cases not operated upon .. 33	26	7	78
Cases operated upon 27	6	21	22
Total 60	32	28	

These figures are striking enough, but we have also to take into consideration the fact that operation has hitherto been reserved as a rule for the worst cases, and often after other forms of treatment have failed. There is thus every reason to hope that when the value of operation is better known, the great majority of the patients will recover, and instead of recovery being the exception, it will become the rule.

There are two methods of treatment by operation:—(1) *Giving rest to the colon by establishing an artificial anus;* (2) *Making an opening through which the colon can be irrigated and the ulcerated areas kept clean,*

Two other methods suggest themselves, namely, to short-circuit the colon by ileo-sigmoidostomy, and to excise the diseased colon. Neither of these is, however, possible except in most exceptional cases. The rectum and sigmoid are generally the parts of the bowel in which there is most ulceration, and therefore the anastomosis would have to be done with diseased bowel. For the same reason excision would not be possible even if the patients were not too ill to stand so severe an operation.

1. GIVING REST TO THE COLON.—As the pathology of ulcerative colitis clearly shows that the ulceration usually extends throughout the whole of the colon, it is obvious that the artificial anus should be made in the cæcum if the operation is to be successful. This is also clearly shown by the results of operation, as out of six cases treated by colostomy on the left side, three died, while the six cases treated by cæcostomy all recovered.

Where right-sided colostomy or cæcostomy has been performed, the results have been good as regards a cure of the ulceration. The symptoms have subsided, and the patient has rapidly improved in health. The operation is, however, objectionable, as a right-sided colostomy is even more unpleasant than a left-sided colostomy. Moreover, it is frequently impossible or inadvisable to close the opening, and it has to be retained as a permanent outlet for the fæces. In several cases an attempt to close the opening has immediately resulted in a recurrence of the symptoms of ulceration, and in a few, fatal peritonitis has resulted from the attempt. Mr. Makins,[*] who has performed the operation in six cases, has given it as his opinion that if the opening cannot be closed in eight or nine months, it will subsequently become impossible to close it on account of the contraction which occurs in the disused colon, and that if a right-sided colostomy is performed in these cases the patient must be prepared for the probability that the opening will be a permanent one.

Therefore, as regards curing the patient, a right-sided colostomy may be expected to give good results; but it will not infrequently be at the expense of leaving the patient with a permanent artificial anus. A right-sided lumbar colostomy is preferable to a cæcostomy on account of the more solid nature of the stools, and appears to give as good results as a cæcostomy.

2. OPERATION FOR ESTABLISHING A MEANS OF IRRIGATING THE COLON.—The operation of choice in cases of ulcerative colitis is, without doubt, appendicostomy, or if this is impossible owing to the appendix being diseased or having already been removed, a valvular opening which will just admit a catheter should be established. At first the colon should be washed out twice

---

[*] *Proc. Roy. Soc. of Med.* Jan. 26, 1909, Med. Sect.

daily with either plain water or normal saline, a tube being placed through the anal sphincters to allow the fluid to run out. Later, a weak solution of protargol or argyrol may be used with advantage.

This operation gives excellent results; the ulceration, as a rule, quickly heals, the patient puts on weight, and the diarrhœa is controlled.

I have seen most excellent results from this operation in bad ulcerative colitis, and it has such manifest advantages over colostomy that I think it should always be done except, perhaps, in a few exceptional cases. It does not leave the patient with an unpleasant opening, or cause him the least discomfort or inconvenience, and it can be closed at any time without an operation.

The following are instances of the good results which follow this operation :—

Case.—The patient was a man, aged 35, who for nine months had been suffering from almost constant diarrhœa. He was very weak and much wasted. The stools contained a considerable quantity of blood. A sigmoidoscopic examination showed numerous discrete ulcers in the pelvic colon. Appendicostomy was performed, and the colon kept washed out with warm water. The diarrhœa was at once controlled, there was no further bleeding, and the patient made a rapid recovery. A month after the operation he left the hospital. He continued for six months to wash the colon out daily, but returned to his employment. He had no further symptoms, and a sigmoidoscopic examination six weeks after operation showed that all the ulcers were healed. A year and three months after operation he was quite well and had had no recurrence of the previous symptoms.

Case.—A lady, aged 25, had for five weeks been suffering from constant diarrhœa, and the symptoms, in spite of all treatment, had been getting worse during the last month. The stools contained large quantities of blood, she had become very anæmic, and wasted almost to a skeleton. Some six months previously she had had a slight similar attack, which had, however, quickly passed off. On the present occasion, however, she had become steadily worse, and her condition was very grave. The sigmoidoscope showed extensive ulceration and a hæmorrhagic condition of the mucous membrane. Treatment by a special vaccine failed to do any good. Appendicostomy was performed, and the colon was washed out frequently with warm water. As a result of this treatment the hæmorrhage and diarrhœa were controlled within thirty-six hours. The patient rapidly improved in health, and in two months was quite well. The irrigation was continued once daily for the next two months.

Case.—I was consulted by a lady, aged 31, who three years ago had contracted dysentery while resident in the East. She had suffered on and off ever since from diarrhœa and bleeding from the bowel. When I saw her the bowels acted six or seven times a day, there was blood in the stools, and she was often sick. Medical treatment had quite failed to do any good, and she was practically confined to bed, the least attempt to move about bringing on severe diarrhœa. Appendicostomy was performed, and at the operation a number of chronic ulcers could be felt in the colon, especially in the transverse portion. The bowel was kept washed out, and in three weeks all the symptoms had disappeared. She became quite well, and was able to return to the East. I have since heard from her, and there has been no return of the symptoms.

Of the 18 cases which I have been able to collect in which appendicostomy was performed, 17 recovered, and 8 of these remained well and free from any relapse. One died a year later from the results of another operation, though there was no return of the ulceration. One died three weeks after the operation, but it was found post mortem that the lower part of the ileum was ulcerated in addition to the colon.

Appendicostomy and irrigation of the colon appears to be the best treatment in these cases. It should be performed as soon as possible, and not as a last resort.

Treatment of Complications.

Of these there are three which are likely to call for surgical treatment: (1) *Perforation;* (2) *Hæmorrhage;* (3) *Abscess.*

1. PERFORATION.—With very few exceptions this complication is fatal, unless an operation can be performed in time; and only immediate intervention can save the patient's life.

The success which has attended the treatment by operation of perforated gastric ulcer, and perforation of the appendix, can certainly be repeated in dealing with these cases of perforating ulcer of the colon, once the condition becomes sufficiently well recognized for an early diagnosis to be made, and providing the surgeon is able to operate soon after the perforation has taken place. Unfortunately, up to the present, this has seldom been the case; the perforation has either not

ULCERATIVE COLITIS

been diagnosed during life, or the surgeon has been called in too late for there to be any reasonable chance of doing good.

A correct diagnosis is very difficult in these cases, and it will seldom be possible for the clinician to do more than diagnose a probable perforation in some part of the intestine. Unless the surgeon bears in mind the possibility of a perforating ulcer of the colon when he comes to operate, and carefully examines the colon after having excluded a perforated appendix or gastric ulcer, the perforation will probably be missed. This occurred in one case where perforation and general peritonitis were diagnosed and the abdomen opened; a slightly inflamed appendix was removed, but the cause of the peritonitis, which was a perforation of the colon at the hepatic flexure, was missed, and the patient died. The difficulty of finding and closing the perforation may be considerable; it may be in any portion of the colon and on any aspect. Moreover, there may be more than one perforation in the same case.

The method of dealing with the perforation will vary with the nature of the case. It may be treated like a perforation of the stomach and closed by a purse-string suture reinforced by a row of Lembert sutures. In one case, a Paul's tube was tied into the perforation, which was in the cæcum, and an artificial anus established. The operation in this case was performed too late, and the patient died. Though this is a rapid method of dealing with the perforation in cases when speed is of the first importance, it is not a satisfactory operation. Another method is to resect the ulcer and close the wound in the bowel in the opposite direction, so as not to narrow the lumen; or, if the ulcer is large, to resect a few inches of the colon and unite the ends.

I have been able to collect 42 cases of perforation of the colon due to simple ulceration. This does not include any cases of perforating false diverticula. All died, with the exception of three. Only six were operated upon, but of these, three recovered. Thus, without operation the mortality would appear to be 100 per cent, and there is no doubt that this mortality can be greatly reduced by operation.

Of the six cases operated upon, the ulcer was missed in the three that died. One was treated by closing the perforation, and recovered. In one, an abscess was opened and a fæcal fistula found; later, the portion of colon (sigmoid flexure) containing the ulcer was successfully resected.

In the third case that recovered, the operation consisted only of opening an abscess. In another, enterotomy was performed, but the patient died, and post mortem a perforating ulcer in the sigmoid was discovered.

2. HÆMORRHAGE.—This is best treated by washing out the bowel with some suitable astringent such as hazeline two drachms to the pint, complete rest, and the administration of opium (see page 167).

3. ABSCESS.—As soon as there is reason to believe that an abscess has formed, an operation should be performed and adequate drainage provided for.

REFERENCES.

HALE WHITE.—*Guy's Hosp. Rep.* 1888.
NOTHNAGEL.—*Diseases of Intestines and Peritoneum.* English edition edited by H. D. Rolleston.
DICKINSON.—*Trans. Path. Soc.* xxxii.
" Discussion on Ulcerative Colitis," *Proc. Roy. Soc. of Med.* Jan. 26, 1909.

Chapter XIII.

PERICOLITIS.

By this is meant a condition of inflammation around the colon, and involving its walls. In many respects it closely resembles perityphlitis or appendicitis, generally differing only in the locality in which it is situated.

It is only of comparatively recent years that pericolitis has been recognized as a definite form of disease, though many observers had previously recorded cases of abscess or inflammatory tumours in connection with the colon. In looking up old records one not infrequently meets with cases which were obviously of this nature, but, as with appendicitis before it became a well-recognized condition, little attention was paid to them, and in very few instances were really careful observations made. They were classed as inflammation of the bowels, post-peritoneal or intra-peritoneal abscess, general peritonitis, etc., without any distinction being made as to the causation or pathology. Isolated specimens are to be found in museums, but in many instances they are wrongly described or classified, and in not a few the specimen is labelled " Cancer of the colon."

Lately more attention has been paid to this disease, and several carefully observed cases have been recorded. Even at the present time, however, pericolitis does not find a place in the ordinary medical text-books, and many medical men know nothing about it, or look upon it only as a rare pathological condition of little interest except to the pathologist.

Pericolitis is probably not a rare condition, but on the other hand it is one which occurs comparatively often, and I believe that, when its symptoms and pathology are well known and recognized, it will be found to be a by no means uncommon disease of the alimentary tract.

Post-mortem statistics would lead us to conclude that pericolitis is a rare disease. Cases are very difficult to find in the post-mortem records of large hospitals, and the same applies to the hospital case-books. If classified at all, it is under the general head of abscess, and usually the cause is not even suggested.

The great majority of cases have ended fatally, and the condition has only been detected post mortem.

Etiology.

Pericolitis is a disease of advanced life. The majority of the patients are over the age of forty, the average of the cases I have been able to collect being fifty years. The youngest I have found is that of a girl of eighteen. There are two others of twenty-two and one of twenty-three in my series, but most are considerably older.

It is somewhat remarkable that, apart from tubercle, there appear to be no records of the condition in children, although intestinal complaints are common enough in infancy. The reason why the disease is chiefly confined to the later part of life lies probably in the important part played by chronic constipation as an etiological factor.

The portion of the colon most commonly attacked in pericolitis is the sigmoid flexure, but any part may be affected. In the great majority of cases the condition occurs either in the sigmoid flexure or lower part of the descending colon. In a few the splenic angle has been the site of the disease, and I have been able to find two instances only of the transverse colon being affected.

Pericolitis, like all forms of inflammation, may be either acute or chronic, but except in relation to the symptoms, such a classification is of little if any value, and the cases will therefore be arranged on a pathological basis. The term is a wide one and covers a number of pathological conditions, or rather there are many such conditions which may give rise to pericolitis. Many cases have been described as pericolitis sinistra, perisigmoiditis, and diverticulitis; but there is no advantage in using these names: the term pericolitis includes them, and the condition does not differ in any important particular when it occurs in different parts of the colon.

Under the general heading we should include most of the cases of tuberculosis of the colon, and certainly all those of hyperplastic tuberculosis. Most cases of cancer of the colon are also sooner or later complicated by a pericolitis, and it is necessary, therefore, to include this form of the condition. As, however, the subjects of tuberculosis of the colon and of cancer are more conveniently considered elsewhere, these two conditions will not be included here.

It is obvious that with the exception of those cases in which septic infection has spread to the bowel wall from some source unconnected with the colon, there must be a lesion of the wall of the colon which allows infective material to escape from the bowel lumen. In other words, there must be either a perforation of the colon or an infiltration of its wall by some infective process before pericolitis can occur. In the order of their importance in producing pericolitis, the causes are as follows : (1) *Diverticula of the colon;* (2) *Ulceration;* (3) *Perforation by foreign bodies;* (4) *Tubercle;* (5) *Cancer;* (6) *Syphilis;* (7) *Traumatism.*

1. DIVERTICULA OF THE COLON.—By far the most important cause of pericolitis is the formation of acquired diverticula.

Since attention was first attracted to the presence of these diverticula they have been a source of much interest to surgeons and pathologists, and it is now becoming evident that they are by no means as rare as was at first supposed.

They consist of small pouches or hernial protrusions of the colon, somewhat resembling the pouches seen in the bladders of old men who have had obstructive urinary trouble.

They vary in size, from minute canals which can hardly be detected except by microscopic examination of cut sections of the bowel, to large elongated pouches resembling the vermiform appendix or a Meckel's diverticulum. They are sometimes round, and may be described as resembling cherries, but more often are long finger-like pouches with a somewhat dilated extremity. In one of my cases the largest diverticulum was about 2½ inches in length, and about the thickness of a normal appendix vermiformis. It passed down between the layers of the mesosigmoid, and the opening from the bowel, which was at the mesenteric attachment of the sigmoid, easily admitted a large-sized probe. In many cases, however, they are much shorter than this, and will admit only a bristle with difficulty.

The commonest situation for diverticula is near the mesenteric attachment of the bowel ; but they may occur at any position between the longitudinal muscle-bands. They may be found

PERICOLITIS

on the free edge of the bowel almost opposite the mesenteric attachment. It is not uncommon to find one of them passing into an appendix epiploica, and several writers have concluded that these diverticula are simply hollow appendices epiploicæ which communicate with the bowel lumen. This is certainly not the case, as the normal appendices epiploicæ are simply small accumulations of the sub-peritoneal fat or sub-peritoneal

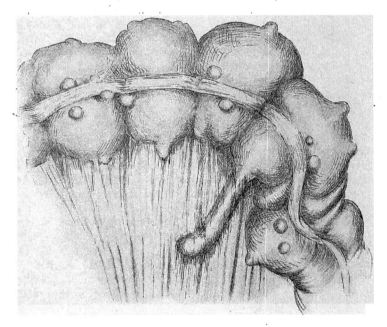

Fig. 47.—Drawing of the pelvic colon in a man, aged 62, showing numerous diverticula. One large diverticulum passed down between the layers of the mesosigmoid; its extremity was dilated and contained a stercolith.

lipomata, and have no connection whatever with the muscular coat of the bowel, and certainly not with the mucous membrane. The diverticula on the other hand, are direct protrusions from the bowel lumen, and the fact that they may sometimes be found passing into an appendix epiploica must, I think, be looked upon as merely a fortuitous circumstance.

They occur at just the positions where the appendices are

commonly found, and it is probable that in seeking a line of least resistance in which to extend their growth they readily find their way into the appendices. In point of fact they are frequently found to lead into the appendices, and they then become distended into a bulbous end which remains connected to the bowel lumen by a narrow channel. Not infrequently they push down between the layers of the mesosigmoid, and may then reach a considerable length.

In Charing Cross Hospital Museum there is a beautiful specimen of a colon showing these diverticula occupying the appendices epiploicæ. They open into the bowel lumen between the valvulæ conniventes by openings which, in most cases, will admit the tip of the little finger. The ends of the diverticula are dilated into pouches occupying the appendices epiploicæ. Most of the fat previously present in the appendices has been absorbed, but in some of them a thin layer of fat still remains separating the diverticulum from the peritoneal covering. In this specimen there appears to be very little thickening or inflammation around the colon.

These diverticula are true protrusions of the bowel; and at first, and before secondary changes have occurred in them, all the coats of the colon are represented in their walls, except occasionally the muscular coat. Presumably, when the muscular coat is not represented, the pouching has occurred between the fasiculi of the muscle, and thus has not carried the muscular coat with it. In a considerable number, however, the muscular coat can be demonstrated in the wall of the diverticulum. As it enlarges, and as secondary inflammatory changes occur in its walls, any muscular tissue atrophies, so that, in the later stages, no trace of any muscular tissue can be detected.

Edel has demonstrated the presence of a muscular coat to be quite frequent on microscopical examination, and this was also shown in one of Moynihan's cases. In one of my own cases the remains of the muscular coat could be clearly seen on microscopical examination.

The diverticula are always lined by mucous membrane, though this may be much changed from secondary inflammation. There is usually a thick layer of fibrous tissue in their walls, due mostly to inflammation. Outside they are covered by peritoneum, and if they have passed into an appendix, there may be a layer of fat.

PERICOLITIS

They would appear from post-mortem statistics to be very rare, out of 12,115 necropsies collected from three hospitals, diverticula of the colon were only present in 28. But it is highly probable that they are nothing like so rare as these figures seem to show. I have been able to find 58 cases. Graser, who examined microscopically the sigmoid flexures from 28 bodies of elderly persons, found small diverticula in 10.

They may be either congenital or acquired, but are certainly an acquired condition in the vast majority of cases. This is shown by the fact that pericolitis due to diverticula apparently does not occur in childhood, but on the other hand is chiefly confined to elderly people. I have been entirely unable to find a single instance by examining the colons of children and infants.

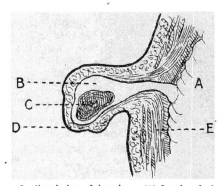

Fig. 48.—Diagram of a diverticulum of the colon. (A) Interior of colon. (B) Cavity of diverticulum. (C) Stercolith. (D) Appendix epiploica. (E) Muscular coat of colon.

Diverticula are not peculiar to the colon, but may occur in the small intestine, apart from Meckel's diverticulum. They are not found in the cæcum, and but rarely in the ascending and transverse colon. The commonest situation is in the lower part of the descending colon, and more especially in the sigmoid flexure.

They never occur in the rectum, probably because of the thicker muscular coat of the latter viscus.

They may be single, but in most cases are multiple. In many of the cases great numbers of these diverticula are present.

It is interesting to notice that in a case recorded by Rolleston there was a pressure diverticulum of the pharynx in addition to diverticula in the sigmoid flexure. Acquired diverticula of the colon generally contain fæcal material: in fact one might say that they invariably do ; and it is to their contents rather than to themselves that they owe their pathological significance. In many cases the fæcal material has become hardened from long residence within the pouch, and has formed a concretion or stercolith. In one of my cases the concretion was of the size and consistence of a date-stone. They are generally found in the pouched extremity of the diverticulum.

The cause of the formation of these diverticula has been the subject of considerable discussion ; but there is little doubt they are simply pressure herniæ of the mucous membrane, produced in most cases by old-standing constipation.

The youngest case in which they have been found is Fielder's, of a patient aged 22. In most the subjects are elderly. In 80 cases collected by Telling, the average age was 60, and in my series, is about the same. This, and the fact already referred to, that post mortem they are not found in children, but only in adults, and chiefly in elderly adults, point to some long-continued cause, associated probably with weakening of the musculature of the gut-wall from atrophy.

The fact that chronic constipation is present in most of the cases in which diverticula are found, combined with the other fact that they are commonest in the sigmoid flexure, which we know to be the chief receptacle for fæcal material, and certainly that portion of the bowel in which the contents are longest retained, seems to support the view that constipation is an important etiological factor. But it must not be forgotten that constipation is very common without the formation of diverticula. Also, if constipation were the only cause, we should expect to find diverticula more frequently present in women than men ; but the reverse is apparently the case. While, therefore, it cannot be doubted that constipation is an important factor, there must be some other cause to account for their formation.

A fact of some importance, first noticed by Klebs, is that the commonest situation for the diverticula is along the edge of the mesenteric attachment, which is also the position at which the blood-vessels of the gut pierce the muscular coat. These are obviously points of weakness in the bowel wall, but on the other hand many of the diverticula occur on the convexity of the bowel, where there are no vessels entering.

I think the probable explanation of the formation of these pouches is that they are true pressure-herniæ through a weakened muscular wall produced by chronic constipation. They are a kind of exaggeration of the normal sacculi of the colon occurring between the longitudinal muscle-bands. That pressure is not the sole cause is evident from the fact that they are not commonly found above a stricture of the rectum, as one would otherwise expect.

I have seen one case in which a large diverticulum was present in the upper part of the sigmoid above a rectal stricture

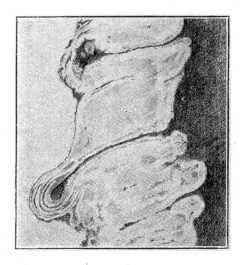

Fig. 49.—Section of the wall of the colon in a case of pericolitis due to multiple diverticula.

(carcinoma) ; but although I have collected a large number of cases of these diverticula, I have found no other such instance.

Pathological Changes in Acquired Diverticula of the Colon which may cause Pericolitis.—The pathological conditions which may occur in one of these diverticula are practically identical with those which may occur in the vermiform appendix.

Once formed, the pouch tends to enlarge and to elongate beneath the peritoneum. Fæcal material will find its way into it, but will not readily get out again, with the result that a concretion is soon formed. The muscular coat, if present, soon

PERICOLITIS

atrophies and the mucous membrane becomes thinned or ulcerated, so that in their later stages the pouches have very thin walls consisting of little more than peritoneum. As with the appendix, the presence of the fæcal concretion readily sets up ulceration in the interior of the diverticulum, and we thus have inflammation of the wall of the diverticulum, and all the factors necessary for the production of an abscess or perforation.

Perforation may result either from sloughing of the concretion through the walls of the diverticulum (and in one or two cases the concretion has been found loose in the peritoneal cavity), from gangrene of the diverticulum, or from the formation of a local abscess which has subsequently burst into the peritoneal cavity. Examples of all these conditions are to be met with.

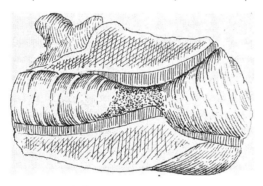

Fig. 50.—Tuberculous pericolitis producing a stricture. The stricture is ulcerated, and the colon above dilated.

Occasionally a chronic pericolitis is set up which results in the formation of a dense mass of fibrous tissue around the diverticula, protecting them from perforating, but causing a dense cicatricial mass which may result in obstruction of the bowel, and which may closely simulate malignant disease. Apart from the presence of concretions, diverticula may contain foreign bodies, and two cases are recorded by Bland Sutton of an inflamed diverticulum of the sigmoid which contained a piece of straw.

Several illustrations of diverticula and of their microscopic appearance are appended.

In one of the cases, a diverticulum of the cæcum had become

infected with tubercle and caused tuberculous ulceration of the ascending colon.

2. ULCERATION.—Any form of ulceration of the colon may cause pericolitis. The ulcers may be either single or multiple. They are generally of old standing, and have either perforated the bowel-wall or are covered on the outer side by peritoneum only. They are often cratiform, and the colon at the base of the ulcer has become adherent to other structures, or is densely matted over with fibrous tissue. In one of my cases in which the mucous membrane of the sigmoid was extensively ulcerated, the bowel-wall was so thick and hard as to suggest at first that it was the site of an infiltrating carcinoma, which view was apparently supported by the presence of numerous enlarged glands in the mesosigmoid. A careful examination, however, showed that the thickening of the bowel-wall was entirely secondary to the ulceration, and that the gland enlargement was inflammatory.

3. PERFORATION BY FOREIGN BODIES.—These may be either pins, fish-bones, or other sharp bodies which have been swallowed, or foreign bodies introduced into the rectum. A case was recently reported in one of the medical journals, of a girl who had swallowed a packet of needles; several of these were found to have reached the colon and perforated its walls, producing local adhesions and inflammation, but without causing a general peritonitis.

A case is recorded by Cuff, in which a piece of straw, used by the patient for picking his teeth, was swallowed and perforated the colon. A chronic pericolitis occurred, and a hard mass formed in the abdomen and became adherent to the abdominal wall, and discharged pus. The pus was found on examination to contain the ray fungus: so that in this case the pericolitis was due to actinomycosis.

4, 5. TUBERCLE AND CANCER.—These causes of pericolitis will be considered in detail in Chapters XIV and XVIII.

6. SYPHILIS.—This does not appear to be a usual cause of pericolitis. It is mentioned, however, by one or two writers on the subject, and Cavaillon and Bardin have recorded four cases.

7. TRAUMATISM.—The colon is not readily subject to injury from direct violence, and it is difficult to prove that a pericolitis has arisen directly as the result of an injury. In two cases recorded by D'Arcy Power, there was a definite history of abdominal traumatism. In one, a woman had been kicked

in the abdomen, and in the other the patient had been struck in the abdomen while at work.

In one or two other instances there are also histories of abdominal injury, but in none of them was any tear or injury of the colon demonstrated.

Symptoms.

These vary greatly, according to the cause of the condition and the degree of inflammation present. From a clinical point of view we may distinguish two distinct types : cases in which there is tumour formation, and those in which there is abscess. Thus in many patients the condition first draws attention to itself by the presence of a tumour in the abdomen, in others by signs of an intra-abdominal abscess, or by perforation and general peritonitis, while in a few the onset of intestinal obstruction is the first evidence of anything being wrong.

Interest has chiefly centred round those cases in which a tumour forms in some part of the colon, as these tumours so closely simulate cancer of the bowel that they are usually mistaken for it. It is interesting in this connection to notice that many cases of supposed spontaneous disappearance, or cure without operation, of cancer of the bowel, are without doubt in reality pericolitis in which the tumour has been mistaken for cancer.

These tumours are due to thickening of the bowel-wall from chronic inflammation. They grow slowly, and are often very hard, due to the deposit of fibrous tissue, so that it is usually impossible from the symptoms to distinguish them from malignant disease. Short of a microscopical examination, they cannot be diagnosed from cancer except in a few instances where the history may assist us, as in the following case :—

Case.—The patient was an elderly lady whom I saw in consultation with her medical attendant with a view to the possibility of closing a colotomy opening of five years' standing. There was a history that about six years ago she commenced to have great difficulty in getting the bowels open. This gradually increased until it terminated in an attack of acute intestinal obstruction. For the relief of this a left inguinal colotomy was performed, and at the operation a large, hard, nodular tumour was discovered in the sigmoid flexure. This tumour was diagnosed as a large inoperable cancer, and the patient was not expected to live more than a few months. After the operation she got better, and had no symptoms beyond those occasioned by the inconvenience of the colotomy opening. At the time I saw her, five years after the operation, she was in good health, and as some fæcal material passed by the anus it was hoped that the colotomy opening might be closed. A sigmoidoscopic examination showed the rectum and lower part of the sigmoid to be normal, but above this the bowel was fixed, and there was a large mass in the bowel wall. From the colotomy opening, a large, hard, nodular mass could be felt in the bowel wall, but not invading the mucosa. It was firmly fixed, and adherent to the left iliac fossa. Just below the colotomy opening there was a tight stricture of the colon which would barely admit the tip of my index finger. The patient had never passed any blood, or experienced any symptoms pointing to ulceration of the mucosa. There is little doubt that this was a case of chronic pericolitis, due probably to diverticula.

In the more acute cases, where there is abscess formation, the symptoms are exactly the same as those of appendicitis, except that the situation is different. Several of these have been described as appendicitis on the left side of the abdomen. There is a high or intermittent temperature, with rigors and sweats; pain, localized to some part of the colon, and local peritonitis. A tender swelling may be present, and there may be fluctuation in this on careful palpation. The abdominal wall is rigid, and the patient lies with the legs drawn up and in considerable pain. If perforation has occurred, the usual symptoms of commencing general peritonitis will show themselves. An exact diagnosis is seldom possible, but when we see a patient with all the symptoms of appendicitis, but with the signs localized to some other part of the abdomen than the appendix region, we should be suspicious of this condition.

The following is a good instance of pericolitis with perforation :

Case.—A caretaker, aged 57, was admitted to St. George's Hospital with symptoms of acute general peritonitis. There was a history of sudden abdominal pain following a dose of castor oil. On opening the abdomen it was found that the appendix was not the cause of the peritonitis, but the colon in the left iliac fossa was bound down by adhesions and was perforated. The abdomen was drained, but the patient died in a few hours. The autopsy revealed old adhesions and thickening of the pelvic colon, and a diverticulum which had perforated into the peritoneal cavity. There were numerous diverticula throughout the colon.

The following, which is a good instance of pericolitis with

abscess formation, is recorded by Mr. D'Arcy Power (*Brit. Med. Journ.* Nov. 3rd, 1906) :—

Case.—The patient, a married woman, aged 38, was admitted to the Bolingbroke Hospital, complaining of pain and a lump in her stomach. There was a history of her having been kicked in the abdomen on several occasions. Ten days before admission she was seized with severe abdominal pain quite suddenly while at work. During the following week the pain continued, and on one occasion she vomited. The bowels were, however, relieved daily. At the end of the week she suddenly became worse, and her temperature rose. On admission, her pulse was 128 and her temperature 102° F. The left side of the abdomen was rigid and tender, and a tumour could be felt to the left of and above the umbilicus. The abdomen was resonant over the swelling. A blood-count showed a marked leucocytosis.

The abdomen was opened over the swelling, and a large abscess was found extending backwards to the posterior abdominal wall, and downwards along the inner side of the descending colon. The abscess was drained, and the patient made a good recovery.

THE PATHOLOGICAL CONDITIONS ARISING FROM PERICOLITIS.

Pericolitis may give rise to any of the following pathological conditions : (1) *Tumour or swelling ;* (2) *Abscess ;* (3) *Stricture of the colon ;* (4) *Adhesions to other organs ;* (5) *Fistulæ ;* (6) *Vesico-colic fistulæ ;* (7) *Cancer ;* (8) *General peritonitis ;* (9) *Deformities and contractions of the mesosigmoid.*

1. **Tumour Formation.**—Chronic pericolitis may result in the formation of a tumour which to the naked eye is indistinguishable from a malignant growth, and in many instances it has only been on microscopical examination that the true pathology of the condition has been detected.

The tumour is usually very hard, irregular in shape, and adherent to neighbouring structures. The lymphatic glands draining the affected area are usually enlarged.

On examination after removal, either as the result of an operation or "post mortem," evidence of inflammation is usually noticed. The mass may be red and œdematous in places, while here and there white patches of lymph can often be seen, which mark the site of recent adhesions to neighbouring structures. The peritoneum is usually rough and much thickened. When cut open the walls are seen to be thickened and indurated, and to the naked eye may closely resemble a malignant growth. In some instances the wall of the bowel has been an inch or two in thickness, and intensely hard. Thickening is due to inflammatory infiltration of all the coats of the bowel, and subsequent formation of fibrous tissue. In fact the entire bowel-wall may be converted into a solid mass of fibrous tissue over an inch in thickness. The thickening is not confined to any one aspect of the bowel-wall, but in most cases completely surrounds it, though it is often considerably greater in one part than another. The mucous membrane may be almost unaffected, and on examination be quite smooth; in this respect it differs markedly from the condition usually seen in cancer. The presence of diverticula or ulcers may often be detected on careful examination, as the condition has generally arisen from some cause within the bowel.

There is often narrowing of the bowel lumen at the site of the tumour, and this may have resulted in secondary ulceration in the bowel *above* the stricture from fæcal retention. This, however, must not be confused with the primary cause of the condition.

The stricture itself is a secondary result of the formation and subsequent contraction of the fibrous tissue in the wall of the colon, and in this respect closely resembles the formation of the typical ring stricture often seen in cancer of the colon. There may be only a ring stricture, or in some cases a long narrow canal is formed. In some, the lumen has been so narrowed as barely to admit a lead pencil. In others, however, considerable tumour formation occurs, with but little narrowing of the bowel lumen.

Curiously enough, the mucous membrane may not be involved at all in the inflammatory process, even though apparently the condition has arisen from some defect in the mucous lining of the canal. Thus in one case, although a considerable tumour existed, and the walls of the bowel were over half-an-inch thick, the mucosa showed no changes, and moved freely on the subjacent coat.

The thickened walls of the bowel may show necrotic or breaking down areas, but this is the exception rather than the rule. Careful examination of the walls of the bowel after it has been cut open will not infrequently reveal the presence of diverticula or pouches, usually multiple, and often very narrow.

PERICOLITIS

Microscopical Appearances.—The tumour is generally seen to consist mainly of a dense mass of fibrous tissue and round-celled infiltration, quantities of round cells being interspersed here and there throughout the mass. At the areas of more active or recent inflammation the ordinary appearances of chronic inflammation may be seen, namely, loose connective tissue crowded with lymphocytes. Areas containing necrotic tissue or blood extravasation may also be found. The peritoneum shows chronic inflammatory changes, is usually much thickened, and the muscular coat much atrophied. The mucosa often shows comparatively little change, but in some cases is a good deal atrophied, the glandular elements having disappeared.

2. Abscess.—This is a not uncommon result of pericolitis. The abscess may be single, or there may be a large indurated mass containing numerous small abscesses.

These are similar to abscesses accompanying appendicitis, and are usually shut off from the general peritoneal cavity by adhesions to neighbouring coils of bowel. The abscess may be post-peritoneal, in which case it is often very extensive, surrounding the kidney, and passing up to the diaphragm and down into the pelvis. The formation of a post-peritoneal abscess seems to be most often associated with pericolitis of the ascending colon. They may burst externally, or into the bowel, or may rupture into the peritoneal cavity; instances of all these conditions have been met with. Such abscesses are also a not uncommon cause of vesicocolic fistula. As is the case with appendicitis, they may result from an actual perforation of the bowel, or may arise without any perforation being detectable: presumably from the passage of micro-organisms along the lymphatics, or even through the damaged bowel-wall. A common cause is perforation of a false diverticulum of the colon.

In a case recorded by Telling, acute intestinal obstruction had resulted from the small bowel becoming adherent to a mass of pericolitis in the sigmoid flexure. A short-circuiting operation was performed, but the patient died. It was then found that there were several diverticula in the sigmoid, some of which had perforated and caused adhesions to the ileum.

Another case is recorded by Moynihan, in which also the ileum had become adherent to the sigmoid as the result of pericolitis, with resulting acute obstruction. The patient died five days after a double enterotomy had been performed. There is a specimen in Guy's Hospital Museum of a band between the sigmoid flexure and the mesentery of the ileum. The band is formed by two adherent appendices epiploicæ, and there is some thickening of the wall of the sigmoid. The patient died from intestinal obstruction.

Tuttle records a case of chronic obstruction resulting from kinking of the sigmoid flexure due to two appendices becoming adherent to each other as the result of local pericolitis.

3. **Stricture.**—In many instances a fibrous stricture giving rise to obstruction has been the cause of death, or has called for the performance of an operation for its relief. The amount of narrowing of the colon may be very considerable, and as the commonest situation for the condition is in the sigmoid flexure, where the bowel contents are usually solid, obstruction readily occurs.

4. **Adhesions.**—Extensive adhesions of the affected portion of bowel to surrounding structures are the rule in pericolitis, and are nature's method of protecting the patient from the consequences of the condition.

Favel tells of a woman who suffered from persistent pain in the abdomen, which was found on performing laparotomy to be due to extensive adhesions between the ascending colon and the anterior abdominal wall. In another case, in which the patient suffered from constant pain and frequent vomiting, adhesions were found between the ascending colon and the abdominal wall, involving also the uterus. In both cases the adhesions had arisen from a localized pericolitis of the ascending colon.

Intestinal obstruction resulting from adhesions produced by pericolitis may occur, and is generally due to adhesions between the small intestine and the colon.

5. **Fistulæ.**—These may form from the formation of an abscess which opens upon the abdominal wall, producing a cutaneous fistula, or a communication may take place into some other hollow viscus, such as the stomach or small intestine.

6. **Vesico-colic Fistula.**—One would naturally expect pericolitis, when it affects the sigmoid, to be a common cause of adhesions between this viscus and the bladder, with which it is in close contact, and that the subsequent formation of a

fistula between the two would be a not uncommon complication. This was actually present in sixteen of my collected cases.

There is an interesting example in Guy's Hospital Museum. The patient was a man aged 65, who for twelve years had passed flatus " per urethram." More recently fæces had commenced to escape from the urethra. Mr. Bryant performed colotomy, but the patient died. Post mortem a much thickened sigmoid flexure was found, in the walls of which were numerous diverticula. A fistula some two inches in length established communication between the bladder and the sigmoid.

Pericolitis is probably the commonest cause of these fistulæ, as was pointed out by Mr. Harrison Cripps many years ago, when he showed that the cause was inflammatory in 45 cases out of 63, and malignant in only nine, though it seems generally believed that malignant disease is the commonest cause of these fistulæ. Chavannaz, from a study of 95 cases, came to the conclusion that 24 per cent only were due to malignant disease.

Telling, after a careful investigation of the subject, concludes that pericolitis arising from diverticula of the colon is the commonest cause of these fistulæ, and points out that this much improves the prognosis as regards operative interference.

7. **Cancer.**—I have seen one case in which there was a cancer at the recto-sigmoidal junction associated with several large diverticula of the sigmoid, and pericolitis. The greater part of the sigmoid showed considerable simple inflammatory thickening. It was impossible to be certain that the pericolitis was the primary condition, but it appeared probable.

A case was reported by Hochenegg in 1902 of a patient with cancer of the sigmoid flexure. The whole of the sigmoid flexure being the site of numerous diverticula containing fæcal concretions, he assumed the cancer to have arisen from the irritation of the fæcal material in the diverticula. A case in which a carcinoma of the splenic flexure was associated with numerous diverticula in the sigmoid flexure, and in which the appearances of the growth suggested it had arisen from a diverticulum in the splenic flexure, is reported by Telling.

We know that carcinoma of the appendix may occur apparently as the result of chronic inflammation around a retained calculus in the appendix, and it seems equally probable that a similar result may follow a chronic pericolitis from retained fæcal material in a diverticulum of the sigmoid flexure.

8. **General Peritonitis.**—General peritonitis is a common result of pericolitis, and the usual cause of death from this disease. It may result from a direct perforation of the wall of the colon due to ulceration, or to sloughing of the end of a diverticulum of the colon from rupture of a pericolic abscess into the peritoneal cavity. In one case a fæcal concretion was found loose in the peritoneal cavity, and on the anterior aspect of the sigmoid flexure there was a diverticulum which was partly gangrenous.

Most cases of pericolitis which have been left untreated have died of general peritonitis. In some of these it had not been possible to demonstrate any opening through which infection could have reached the peritoneal cavity, and the abscess, if present, was apparently shut off. In these cases we must assume, either that the opening had been overlooked, had been closed again before death, or that the organisms had passed through the walls of the abscess without perforation being present.

9. **Deformities and Contractions of the Mesosigmoid.**—It is obvious that if chronic inflammation occurs in and around the wall of the sigmoid flexure, the mesosigmoid will be liable to be involved in the subsequent contraction caused by organized fibrous tissue. This arises not uncommonly, and the mesosigmoid may be shortened, contracted, or otherwise deformed to a considerable extent as the result of an old-standing perisigmoiditis.

Such contractions may be of no consequence to the function of the bowel, but occasionally may result in kinking or angulation of the sigmoid, or in such impaired mobility that a serious impediment to the passage of the fæces results. In this way actual acute obstruction—or more frequently a chronic obstruction—is produced. This subject has already been considered in dealing with volvulus and angulation of the pelvic colon.

The effect of a meso-sigmoiditis in producing obstruction, twists, kinks, and other deformities has been pointed out by Reis, Tixier, and Riedel. Reis believes that the meso-sigmoiditis is produced by mesenteric diverticula, which have become inflamed, but no direct proof of this point is recorded.

PERICOLITIS

Treatment of Pericolitis.

To judge by the cases I have been able to collect, pericolitis appears to be a very fatal disease, 70 per cent of the patients having died either from general peritonitis, obstruction, abscess, or pyæmia.

This high mortality must not be attributed, however, to surgical failures, as in many cases no operation was performed, but rather to the absence of a correct diagnosis. The successful treatment of pericolitis, like that of appendicitis, depends to a very large extent upon correct and early diagnosis of the condition. The great majority of cases hitherto have been diagnosed only at an operation, or as the result of a post-mortem examination, and the first essential of successful treatment in dealing with this disease is to get it better recognized, and to obtain a reasonable probability of a correct diagnosis, before the case has advanced too far for operation to be attended by a reasonable possibility of success.

Of the 74 cases which I have been able to collect, 35 were not operated upon, and 39 were. Of those that were not operated upon 33 died, and only 2 recovered; while of the cases operated upon 21 recovered and 18 died.

It must, however, be remembered in considering these figures that a diagnosis has seldom been made except as the result of either an operation or a post-mortem examination, and that in consequence there is in all probability an undue proportion of deaths among the unoperated cases.

These, however, show clearly that there is little to be hoped for from purely medical treatment, a view supported by the fact that death has in most cases been due to general peritonitis, a condition not amenable to purely medical treatment. The only hope is clearly in early operative interference. Of the cases operated upon, 18 died, that is to say, there was an operative mortality of 44 per cent. This is high, and should be much reduced, but it is not surprising when we consider that in most instances a correct diagnosis was not made previous to operation.

Also in several cases the operation was merely an exploratory one, and the abdomen was closed without anything being done. Of 5 cases so treated 4 died. Again, in 7, colotomy was performed under the impression that the case was one of inoperable cancer, and of these 4 died.

The accompanying table shows the results of the various operations that have been performed for pericolitis.

Nature of Operation.	No. of Cases.	No. of Deaths.
Exploratory Laparotomy	5	4
Colotomy	7	5
Excision	12	3
Drainage	5	1
Division of adhesions	3	0
Short-circuiting	2	2
Various	5	3

Colotomy failed because in all but one of the cases there was an abscess in connection with the colon, and although the colotomy relieved the obstruction, the abscess remained and caused peritonitis.

Simple drainage appears to have been very successful, as out of 5 patients so treated 4 recovered. These were all cases of a localized abscess in connection with the colon.

Excision of the entire inflamed portion of colon was performed 12 times, with 9 recoveries.

The causes of death after operation were as follows:—

General peritonitis	14 cases
Pyæmia (not due to operation)	1 case
Obstruction (unrelieved)	1 case
Cardiac failure (on eighth day)	1 case

The treatment of pericolitis is practically the same as for appendicitis, and as with the latter condition, the nature of the operation must to a large extent depend upon the exact pathological condition present, and the acuteness or otherwise of the disease.

Very frequently the symptom necessitating immediate operation has been the development of a local or general peritonitis, due either to abscess formation, or to perforation of the bowel into the peritoneal cavity.

LOCALIZED ABSCESS.—The obvious treatment is to open the abscess and adequately drain it, while at the same time preserving as far as possible the natural adhesive barriers protecting the general peritoneal cavity. The abscess may be very extensive, and for adequate drainage to be established it may be necessary to make a counter-opening in the loin.

When dealing with an abscess in the bowel-wall there may be much difficulty in locating it owing to the dense mass of surrounding adhesions. This is well exemplified by several of the cases in which, after an exploratory laparotomy had been performed without any abscess being discovered, the post-mortem examination showed such to have been present.

PERFORATION AND GENERAL PERITONITIS.—In these cases, though a careful toilet of the peritoneum and the establishment of adequate drainage may suffice, it is advisable, if possible, to find, and close by sutures, the perforation in the colon. Where the perforation is due to the rupture or sloughing of a diverticulum, the perforation may not be single, or other diverticula may be so nearly in the same condition as to threaten to perforate. Also when, as often happens, the perforation has occurred in a dense mass of fibrous tissue and adhesions, very great difficulty may be experienced in closing the perforation.

I have been unable to find a single instance of perforating pericolitis, in which the general peritoneal cavity was infected, which has been successfully operated upon. And yet in no less than 20 of the cases, death was directly due to general peritonitis following a perforation of the colon directly into the peritoneal cavity. This is without counting those cases of general peritonitis due to the secondary bursting of an abscess. Perforation has most frequently resulted from the sloughing or rupture of a diverticulum, usually upon the free border of the sigmoid colon.

Intestinal obstruction was the cause of death in 7 cases, and pyæmia in 3.

The best results have been in cases accompanied by tumour formation. The tumour has in almost every instance been diagnosed as carcinoma previous to operation, and in several instances its inflammatory nature has remained undetected until a microscopical examination has been made. Here again we see the importance from the point of view of treatment of a correct diagnosis. The collected cases show clearly that in quite a number of instances the surgeon has abandoned the operation under the impression that he was dealing with a hopeless case of cancer of the bowel; whereas, had he known that he was only confronted with a simple inflammatory tumour, he might have successfully resected it.

Out of 12 cases treated by resection and end-to-end anastomosis, or the establishment of a colotomy, 9 recovered.

Moynihan resected seven inches of the transverse colon for pericolitis, and subsequently anastomosed the ends in one case, and in another resected five inches of the sigmoid flexure. Mayo excised eight inches of the sigmoid in one case, and in another ten inches of the descending colon and sigmoid flexure.

REFERENCES.

ROLLESTON.—*Lancet.* April, 1905.
MOYNIHAN.—*Edin. Med. Jour.* Mar. 1907.
ROBERTS.—*Brit. Med. Jour.* May 26, 1908.
BREWER.—*Amer. Jour. Med. Sci.* Oct. 1907.
SAILLANT.—*Jour. des Praticiens*, July, 1906.
THOMSON.—*Lancet*, Mar. 21, 1908.
TELLING.—*Lancet*, Mar. 21, 1908.

CHAPTER XIV.

TUBERCULOSIS OF THE COLON.

TUBERCULOUS lesions of the colon are not uncommon. Thus Eisenhardt, out of 1,000 tuberculous subjects, found such lesions of the intestine in 56 per cent; in most of these the colon was affected. In all but four of his cases the condition was secondary to phthisis. Similarly, Herscheimer found it present in all but one out of 58 cases of phthisis.

In considering these figures, however, it must be taken into consideration that practically all these patients had either died from, or were under treatment for, phthisis. Also they only refer to the ordinary ulcerative, and usually secondary, form of intestinal tuberculosis. There can be no doubt that this form of ulcerative colitis is a common secondary complication of phthisis, and the infection is probably caused by the sputum which is swallowed.

There are three types of tuberculous disease of the colon :—

(1) Where it forms part of a general or miliary tuberculosis; (2) Tuberculous ulceration; (3) Hyperplastic tuberculosis.

Tuberculous Ulceration of the Colon (Tuberculous Colitis).—In the ulcerative type, the infection is certainly secondary in most cases to tuberculous lesions of the lungs and air-passages, or the higher parts of the alimentary canal, and is due to direct infection of the mucous membrane with tubercle bacilli. I have been unable to find any case of primary tuberculous ulceration of the colon, and it seems probable that it is always a secondary tuberculous manifestation due to direct infection. In not a few cases it is the chief lesion which calls for treatment. In one case it was apparently secondary to tubercle of the genito-urinary tract. Rarely, however, tuberculous ulceration of the colon may exist apart from evidence of general tuberculosis. Cantley has recorded the case of a girl, four years of age, who had been ill for a year. During six months the stools had been frequent, loose, and very offensive, and for two weeks they had contained small black particles of clotted blood. Vomiting occurred daily, but there was practically no abdominal pain or distention, and no fever. She died ; and at the autopsy two tuberculous ulcers, causing stricture, were found in the colon. There were also extensive ulceration of the cæcum and multiple ulcers in the small intestine, with a little adhesive peritonitis at their bases, but no caseous mesenteric glands. A small old caseous nodule was found at the apex of the left lung.

The ulceration in these cases is of the typical tuberculous type, with overhanging edges and a raw, unhealthy base. On microscopic examination, numerous caseating areas can be seen, and tubercle bacilli are present in great numbers. The ulcers are usually multiple, and often extensive, tending to encircle the bowel ; as a rule there is little or no thickening of the bowel-wall, in which respect it differs markedly from the hyperplastic type of lesion.

Secondary deposits of tubercle, and caseation in the mesenteric glands, are common ; though in one case there was no infection of the glands.

The ulcers may occur in any part of the colon, but are most commonly seen in the cæcum and ascending colon. The ulcers may perforate the bowel wall, and cause either abscess, fistula, or general peritonitis. In four of the cases of perforating ulcer of the colon which I collected the ulceration was tuberculous.

A remarkable case is reported by Grey Turner[*] in which tuberculous ulceration of the ascending colon apparently resulted from infection of a false diverticulum of the cæcum. The wall of the diverticulum was infiltrated with tubercle, and the ulceration had extended into the surrounding tissues.

While the formation of a stricture as the result of tuberculous ulceration of the ileum is common, it very rarely occurs in the colon. Fistula formation is, however, not uncommon. The fistula may open on to the skin surface, into another part of the bowel resulting in a short circuit, or into the vagina, rectum, or bladder.

Hyperplastic Tuberculosis of the Colon.—The hyperplastic form is, apparently, in some instances a primary tuberculous lesion ; in most of the recorded cases there were

---

[*] *Lancet Report*, 16, 1905.

no symptoms of tuberculosis elsewhere, and in two or three of them an autopsy was made, and a careful examination failed to reveal any other lesion of the kind. Also in a considerable number of the hyperplastic cases there is no ulceration and the mucous membrane is intact. It is a very disputed point in these cases whether the tubercle bacillus reaches the colon wall from the bowel lumen or by the blood-stream.

Hyperplastic tuberculosis of the colon is definitely a surgical disease, as it gives rise to tumour formation and stricture of the bowel, and the only rational treatment is by operation.

It has been repeatedly mistaken for cancer, which in symptomatology it closely resembles; but has seldom been diagnosed previous to operation, and often only then after a microscopical examination.

The lesion is very rare; there is not a single specimen in the Royal College of Surgeons Museum, and it is not mentioned in most surgical or medical text-books.

This peculiar form of intestinal tuberculosis was first described in detail by Hartman and Pilliet in 1891. It is of particular interest for two main reasons: First, that it is a manifestation of tubercle quite unlike the lesions usually met with in other organs; secondly, because it is quite commonly mistaken for carcinoma of the bowel. In fact, there is little doubt that a great many of the cases of supposed cancer of the bowel which have got well without operation, or after such operations as short-circuiting or colotomy, were really cases of this disease. They will, however, be referred to again later.

There is much difficulty in studying this disease, as it is hardly yet recognized generally, and consequently cases are often described under some other heading, or simply recorded as rare conditions; in many no proper microscopical examination has been made for tubercle bacilli in the tissues. Though the condition is undoubtedly a rare one, I have been able to find many well-authenticated cases.

The disease appears to occur with about equal frequency in the two sexes. Thus, out of my series of 100 cases, 47 were males and 33 females. In Bernay's 71 collected cases there were 40 men and 31 women. Conrath collected 77 cases, and found 36 men and 41 women.

This affection chiefly attacks those in the middle period of life, between 20 and 40 years of age. This corresponds very closely with the average age for phthisis. In my series the average age is 32; the oldest patient is 78 and the youngest 7 years of age.

It is generally localized to one part of the colon; occasionally, however, there are two or three distinct lesions; and in a few very rare cases the whole or a large part of the colon is affected. It may arise in any portion; but by far the commonest situation is the cæcum and lower part of the ascending colon. The appended table shows the distribution in my collected series of 100 cases:—

Sigmoid flexure	6
Cæcum	48
Cæcum and ascending colon	39
Whole colon	4
Cæcum, ascending and transverse colon	3
Total	100

There appears to be no explanation why the cæcum is the most commonly affected portion.

The characteristic feature is the formation of a tumour in some part of the colon, accompanied by stricture of the bowel lumen. The disease is essentially chronic, the inflammation encouraging the formation of fibrous tissue and thickening, rather than caseation or ulceration. In many cases the mucous membrane is quite intact, and there is no sign of ulceration. The bowel-wall, however, becomes in time greatly thickened, with the formation in most cases of a definite tumour. Constriction and stricture of the bowel may ensue and cause intestinal obstruction. Secondary abscess may occur; but this is unusual. Tuberculous peritonitis is likewise uncommon.

The disease differs very much from common tuberculous lesions, and resembles certain rare cases of tubercle of the skin and larynx, and especially those cases of Hodgkin's disease which, post mortem, have been found to be tuberculous.

As a rule there is a single tumour; but in a few cases there have been several. Trendelenburg has reported a case in which there were five distinct strictures of the colon from this cause; and Borch one in which there were four.

Association with other Tuberculous Lesions.—As a rule, the condition of the colon is the only manifestation of tubercle

THE COLON

to be found ; in only twenty-four out of the one hundred cases I have collected was there any evidence of tubercle elsewhere. In several of these it seems almost certain the other lesion was secondary to that in the colon.

Table of 100 cases :—

No other tuberculous lesion	76
Tuberculous cavity in lungs or scars of old phthisis	18
Tuberculous peritonitis	1
Tubercle of tibia	1
,, of genito-urinary tract	2
,, of phalanges	1
Tuberculous ulcer in vagina	1
	100

It seems evident, therefore, that in most of the cases the disease is a primary tuberculous lesion.

When the cæcum is the affected region the appendix is not as a rule primarily involved, though it not infrequently becomes so secondarily.

MORBID ANATOMY.

The most characteristic lesion is the formation of a tumour in some portion of the colon. The most usual situation, if the thickening is localized to one part of the colon, is the cæcum, especially in the neighbourhood of the ileocæcal valve. Sometimes, however, the transverse colon, or sigmoid, have been alone affected. In a case reported by Claude, the ascending and descending colon were affected, but the transverse colon was free.

In others the greater part of the colon has been involved, and in Lartigau's case the greater part of the small intestine as well. Commonly, the affected portions of bowel are matted in a mass of fibrous adhesions and enlarged lymphatic glands, so that often a large tumour is produced.

The most conspicuous feature is the thickening of the colon wall, which is very marked in all cases. In this it differs widely from other forms of tubercle of the bowel, as instead of there being a destruction of tissue with thinning, there is usually no ulceration, but great thickening and new formation. The bowel-wall feels firm and hard, due to infiltration with round cells and the deposit of fibrous tissue. This spreads equally round the circumference of the bowel-wall, so that in extreme cases the bowel is converted into a hard tube almost resembling a gas-pipe; considerable narrowing of the lumen follows as a result of the disease; and in most cases stenosis results, and chronic or acute obstruction. Stenosis is the common feature, and the bowel lumen may be so completely blocked that it cannot be detected post mortem. Even where no definite stenosis is present, the thickening of the bowel-wall ultimately prevents the peristaltic movements from taking place, and obstruction results from this cause.

In addition to the formation of stenosis by hyperplasia of the bowel-wall, narrowing of the lumen may occur from the contraction of ulcers, and from kinking of the bowel by the contraction of adhesions.

Where the stenosis and thickening are local, considerable

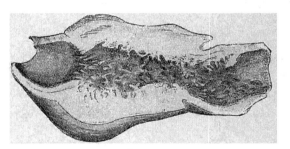

Fig. 51.—Hyperplastic tuberculosis of the colon (*Mr. Nash's case*).

dilatation of the colon above the stricture may occur, and secondary stercoral ulcers may form. Commonly the mucous membrane appears normal and there is no ulceration or breach of the surface. Sometimes the mucous membrane is ulcerated. This is most frequent where there is stricture of the bowel lumen, the ulceration being often confined to the strictured area. This has led some observers to conclude that the stricture is the result of ulceration, which it certainly is not, as some of the cases where there is marked stricture show no ulceration. In many, the ulceration is the ordinary form of septic or traumatic stercoral ulcer found above a stricture of the bowel. In fact, the ulceration, though it may occasionally be tuberculous, is probably most often a secondary result of the stricture.

THE COLON

The mucous membrane is usually thickened, and may show numbers of small tubercles scattered over its surface.

A striking feature in many cases has been the formation of polypoid or papillomatous outgrowths on the mucous membrane. The polypoid growths are usually pedunculated, and hang free in the bowel lumen. Similar sessile tumours are sometimes present in addition, which suggests that this is the early form of the pedunculated polypi. Polypoid growths are often very numerous, and give a most curious appearance to the bowel. They vary in size from quite small round polyps to those as large as hazel-nuts. They are covered over with a layer of

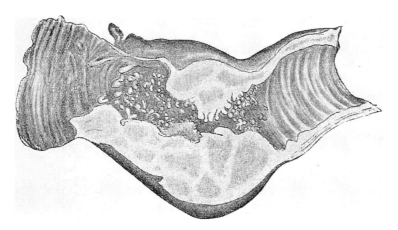

Fig. 52.—Hyperplastic tuberculosis of the colon. The bowel has been cut open longitudinally.

epithelial cells similar to the surrounding mucous membrane, and their centre is continuous with the submucous layer of the bowel-wall, and consists of connective tissue and round-celled infiltration. Occasionally there are caseous foci in the centre of these polypoid growths which may in places have ulcerated through the epithelial layer.

The tumour is very hard and densely indurated. The peritoneum, as a rule, appears normal to the naked eye, though in some cases it is covered with small raised tubercles or nodules of a reddish colour.

If the mass is cut open, the walls of the bowel are seen to be greatly thickened, often to an inch or more, and look and feel like cartilage. The cut section has often a curious bluish-grey translucent appearance, and a glistening surface. The muscular coat is generally much thickened and can be distinctly seen.

Often the greatest thickening is in the subserous layer, which consists of greyish translucent fibrous tissue of cartilaginous hardness, with irregular-shaped areas of yellowish tissue here and there.

The bowel lumen is usually markedly strictured, or there are outgrowths into it. The whole tumour is often very vascular; in some cases it shows areas of degeneration or caseation.

Two types of lesion have been described, the submucous and subserous, according as the thickening and induration are chiefly in the submucous or subserous layers. Both conditions, however, may be seen in the same case, and there seems little advantage in making a distinction between these two forms.

The disease often so closely resembles cancer of the colon that it is only distinguished from it on microscopical examination.

HISTOLOGY.—The mucous membrane often shows little if any change beyond some thickening. Cells undergoing mucoid or cystic degeneration are not infrequently seen. If ulceration is present, the mucous surface presents a mammillated appearance, or is altogether absent.

Polypoid growths, if present, are seen to be outgrowths from the submucosa, and their centres are continuous with it. The epithelium covering them is the same as the normal epithelium, except where ulceration is present, or unless caseation has occurred.

The submucosa is generally markedly thickened by round-celled infiltration and the formation of dense fibrous tissue. Tubercles and giant cells are often to be seen in this layer in considerable numbers. Large polymorphonuclear round cells and coarsely granular eosinophile cells are also to be seen, especially towards the mucous membrane. There may also be caseating tuberculous foci in this layer. The predominating feature is, however, round-celled infiltration with fibrous tissue.

There is always much thickening of the muscular coats, due chiefly to small round-celled infiltration. It is doubtful whether there is really any increase in the number of muscle fibres such as would constitute a true hypertrophy. Some observers claim that there is, while others are equally emphatic that there is not. If dilatation has occurred above the stricture, the muscular coat may be hypertrophied; but apart from this, the hypertrophy appears to be due chiefly to increase in the connective tissue between the fibres.

The subserous layer is often greatly thickened owing to new connective-tissue formation. There is a dense mass of fibrous tissue and small round cells. There are numerous new blood-vessels, often with thick walls.

This layer often contains large vacuolated spaces holding yellow fatty tissue. Giant cells and areas of caseation are much less numerous here than in the submucous layer. The serous layer shows very little change, though it may be much thickened. Tubercle bacilli can usually be found in the submucous layer if sections are carefully stained; compared with other tuberculous lesions, however, they are very scanty. They may be found in large numbers in a section from one part of the tumour, and not at all in a section from another; while in several cases they have been looked for with great care in vain. Portions of the growth have in several instances been inoculated into animals and caused tuberculosis.

Symptoms.

Tuberculous ulceration of the colon gives rise to the ordinary symptoms of ulceration of the bowel, and does not differ in this respect from the non-tuberculous forms of ulcerative colitis. As already stated, it usually occurs as a terminal condition in the later stages of tuberculosis of the lungs. The occurrence of diarrhœa and bloody stools, combined with well-marked signs of phthisis, is indicative of the onset of this condition. Occasionally single ulcers may form and perforate, and in a few instances general peritonitis has occurred from the perforation of a tuberculous ulcer in the colon.

The symptoms of hyperplastic tubercle of the colon are those of a chronic pericolitis. A tumour slowly develops in the abdominal cavity, usually in the cæcal region, and is accompanied by a varying amount of pain and tenderness. In some cases, however, there is little, if any pain, and the tumour is the only sign of anything wrong. Sooner or later the patient either has recurring attacks of partial obstruction, or an acute attack of complete obstruction. In a large number of instances there are symptoms of tuberculosis, either in the lungs or elsewhere, but in about a quarter the condition is apparently primary in the colon.

It is obvious that the symptoms of hyperplastic tubercle of the colon are the same as for cancer of the colon ; and as the latter is the more common disease, it is hardly surprising that the vast majority are diagnosed as cancer.

In hyperplastic tubercle of the colon there is seldom any bleeding ; but in cancer, while bleeding is not invariable, it is usual. The complete absence of blood in the stools, even on microscopical examination, is slightly in favour of tubercle, more especially if the tumour has existed for some time.

Tubercle bacilli can only with difficulty be discovered in sections of the colon wall, and are practically never found in the stools.

SECONDARY LESIONS.—Stricture is an almost invariable accompaniment of the lesion. It is due mainly to the contraction of the fibrous tissue in the bowel wall, and sometimes partly to outgrowths into the lumen. The amount of narrowing of the lumen is often considerable, and the bowel may be almost blocked.

Intestinal obstruction is a common terminal result. As already stated, when ulceration is present it is probably in most cases a stercoral ulceration secondary to the stricture, though sometimes due to caseation of the submucous layer and consequent destruction of the mucous membrane.

Dilatation and hypertrophy of the bowel above the stricture is common, and stercoral ulcers in the dilated portion of bowel have been present in several patients.

In one case recorded by Crowder the tumour had apparently undergone secondary malignant change. It was situate in the cæcum, and presented the typical appearances of hyperplastic tuberculosis with giant cells and tubercle bacilli. In one part the epithelial cells had penetrated to all depths of the tissue, and there were masses of atypical epithelial cells forming tubercles. Apparently the tuberculous lesion was the primary one, and part had undergone secondary malignant change.

The glands are usually enlarged, and show giant cells and caseating areas ; but in several cases there was no gland enlargement. In many, the tumour was tied down by dense adhesions, and, in some, abscess and fistula had formed. These complications, however, generally mark an advanced stage of the disease, when stricture and secondary ulceration have occurred, and are in no way typical of the condition.

The following case is reported by Cumston.*

Case.—The patient was a woman, aged 87, who had complained of pain in the right iliac fossa for eighteen months. She also suffered severely from constipation, and had lost flesh. There was a large mobile tumour in the right side of the abdomen. On opening the abdomen, a tumour in the cæcum was discovered. The cæcum was resected, with 8 cms. of the ileum and 6 cms. of the colon ; the ends were closed, and rejoined by lateral anastomosis. The patient made a good recovery, and was well nineteen months later.

Examination of the specimen showed a cauliflower-like tumour the size of a small apple. On the upper aspect of the ileocæcal valve it completely obstructed the bowel lumen. The cæcal walls were much thickened, and this thickening extended for some distance into the colon. The mucous membrane was intact. There were a few enlarged glands in the mesentery. Microscopical sections of the tumour showed the appearances of tuberculosis.

The following cases were reported by F. S. Kidd :—

Case.—The patient was a girl, aged 7. Three years previously she developed an ulcer in the vagina, which appeared to be tuberculous, and a fæcal fistula formed. Several operations performed with the object of closing this fistula had failed. The abdomen was opened, with the object of performing colotomy, and it was then found that the sigmoid flexure was represented by a hard, indefinite mass about 6 in. long. The whole mass was very vascular. It was diagnosed as cancer, and was brought out of the abdomen, and an artificial anus established. A few days later the growth was cut away. The child recovered with an artificial anus.

Examination of the specimen showed a tight stricture two-and-a-half inches long. There was some ulceration at the site of the stricture, but elsewhere the mucous membrane was normal. The subperitoneal layer of the bowel wall was greatly thickened, and had undergone a curious transformation into pale bluish hyaline tissue almost as hard as cartilage ; in places this was nearly two inches in thickness. Microscopical sections showed fibrillæ, fibroblasts, and round-celled infiltration. There were also numerous large endothelial cells. Sections were stained for tubercle bacilli,

---

* *Annals of Surg.* Nov. 1907.

but they could not be demonstrated; the condition was, however, evidently hyperplastic tuberculosis.

Case.—The patient was a man, aged 57, who died of intestinal obstruction. Post mortem there was a tuberculous scar at the apex of the right lung. At the lower end of the sigmoid flexure there was a hard cartilaginous mass involving the bowel and causing a long narrow stricture. Examination of the tumour showed the mucous membrane to be intact. There were two or three large polypoid masses, which had become impacted in the narrow lumen and caused obstruction. The muscular coat was hypertrophied, and the subperitoneal coat in some places measured as much as three inches in thickness. It was as hard as cartilage. Microscopical sections showed fibrillar tissue and fibroblasts. There was much small-celled infiltration, with numerous large polynuclear cells.

"GAS-PIPE COLON."—There are a few very rare cases of hyperplastic tuberculosis of the colon in which the whole or the greater part is uniformly thickened and densely indurated, and for want of a better term I have called these cases "gas-pipe colon," owing to the resemblance of the bowel to a piece of iron gas-pipe.

I have been able to collect four of these curious cases, one of which I saw myself, and three are from other sources. The close resemblance between the four makes it certain that they were all of the same nature. One was reported as a case of diffuse carcinoma; but it seems certain, from the resemblance to the others and from the fact that symptoms had existed for fourteen years, that it was really hyperplastic tuberculosis.

In my case the patient was a lady, aged 72, who was supposed to be suffering from intestinal obstruction due to cancer of the rectum; some resistance could be felt high up in the bowel. On opening the abdomen to perform colotomy, it was discovered that the entire large bowel, from the rectum to the cæcum, consisted of a hard tube with non-collapsible walls, resembling more than anything else a piece of iron gas-pipe. The colon was diminished in size, being barely an inch in diameter in many places. It was bound down to the posterior wall of the abdomen, and everywhere quite immovable. The walls of the colon were as hard as stone, and nodular. The peritoneal surface of the bowel was covered over with small pink tubercles, and there was much ascites. The wall of the cæcum was greatly thickened; but not in the same way as the rest of the bowel. The lumen was evidently patent, because the bowels had acted occasionally for some weeks, and slightly the day before the operation. The small bowel was normal.

Colotomy could not be performed; but a Paul's tube was tied into the cæcum with difficulty. The patient died, but no post-mortem was obtainable.

The most complete case is Lartigau's. The patient was a man, aged 49, who died after a three years' illness. The thickening of the bowel wall commenced in the upper third of the ileum, and extended throughout the colon to the commencement of the sigmoid flexure. The wall of the bowel was 2·7 cms. thick, and uniform throughout. The lumen was patent, and contained numerous papillomatous masses. Microscopical sections of the bowel wall revealed fibrous thickening, and sections stained for tubercle bacilli showed them to be present in large numbers. There was no ulceration of the mucosa.

C. Briddon's case[*] was that of a man, aged 34, who for twelve years had been suffering from constipation, painful defæcation, and occasional bleeding and tenesmus. This condition had continued with exacerbations. When admitted to the hospital he had six to eight stools daily, which contained blood and mucus and were offensive. Per rectum an indurated mass could be felt. An attempt was made to perform a left inguinal colotomy, but the colon was found to be generally infiltrated and bound down, so that it was impossible to bring any portion of it into the abdominal wound. An incision was made on the right side, but it was found that the whole colon was similarly infiltrated and fixed. The small intestine was normal, and enterotomy was performed. The whole colon was uniformly thickened, and the thickening terminated in a hard cartilaginous mass at the lower end of the sigmoid flexure. The colon was covered with pinkish-coloured nodules, looking like boiled sago.

In J. W. Elliott's case,[†] the patient, a woman, had suffered from constipation and dyspepsia for twelve years. She was admitted into the hospital for a supposed tumour in the rectum. On opening the abdomen it was discovered that the whole colon

---

[*] *Trans. New York Surg. Soc.* May 23, 1894.
[†] *New York Med. Rec.* July 30, 1904.

from the rectum to the splenic flexure was a solid tube so fixed that it could hardly be moved. A right-sided colotomy was performed, and a portion of the mass was removed for examination. It was found to consist of simple inflammatory tissue. Tubercle bacilli were not looked for.

Treatment.

As already stated, the ulcerative form of tubercle of the colon usually occurs as a terminal complication in advanced phthisis, and there is little possibility of treating it, either by medical or surgical means. Occasionally it may happen that surgical treatment is called for to deal with some serious complication which has resulted from the ulceration, such as intractable diarrhœa, perforation with general peritonitis, and abscess. Colotomy can seldom be of any use in treating the diarrhœa, for the cæcum is almost invariably involved. Appendicostomy might be of value in controlling the diarrhœa, by enabling the colon to be washed out periodically, and it has the advantage that it is an operation of so little severity that it could easily be performed in cases where the patient is seriously ill with phthisis, without grave risk. I do not, however, know of any case in which it has been done.

The Treatment of Hyperplastic Tuberculosis of the Colon.—This condition is so rare and so little known, that it is very seldom a correct diagnosis is made previous to operation. The abdomen is generally opened to relieve obstruction, or to explore a tumour, supposed to be malignant. Even when the tumour is seen, it is still usually thought to be malignant; and, indeed the diagnosis cannot be made without cutting open the tumour, or microscoping a portion of it.

This being the case, the treatment adopted is almost invariably that for cancer. It is therefore a fortunate circumstance that the best treatment for hyperplastic tuberculosis is the same, namely excision or short-circuiting. Unfortunately, however, with many patients the tumour is not excised, because the surgeon believes the condition to be one of malignant disease, inoperable because of adhesions and gland involvement; whereas, did he know that it was tubercle, a successful excision might be performed.

Operation is certainly the only cure for this form of tuberculosis of the colon, and medical treatment cannot be expected to do any good, though it may be useful after operation in preventing further tuberculous mischief.

Of my collected series of 100 cases, all but 7 were operated upon, the methods of procedure being as follows :—

Operation.	No. of Cases.	Recovered.	Died.	Mortality per cent.
Resection	63	47	16	25·4
Short-circuiting	16	13	3	18·7
Exclusion with colotomy	7	1		85
Exclusion with lateral anastomosis	3	1	2	66
Totals	89	62	27	

In addition to the above, exploratory laparotomy was performed in four instances. In some of the cases most complicated operations were done, five and even six being performed on the same case at different times.

It will be seen that the lowest operation mortality was obtained by short-circuiting the tumour. This is, however, not so satisfactory as resection, as it leaves a source of infection behind. In several cases the tumour diminished in size, and in some it disappeared after it had been short-circuited. In four, however, a fæcal fistula was left communicating with the tumour; in two, the patient was only slightly improved by the operation; and in another he died soon afterwards from phthisis. Short-circuiting is probably the best operation when resection of the tumour would be attended by considerable risk; but these cases show that resection is a much preferable procedure.

There are seven cases in which, after resection, the ends of the bowel were brought out. In four of these the patient had a permanent fæcal fistula, which could not be closed in spite of secondary operations. Resection of the tumour is certainly the ideal method for this condition, and the operation-mortality is not much higher than that for short-circuiting. It is certain that this mortality of 25 per cent can be considerably lowered by not performing immediate resection and anastomosis where there is obstruction, or the bowel above the tumour cannot be emptied previous to operation.

The following table shows the methods adopted in dealing with the ends of the bowel after resection :—

	Cases.	Deaths.	Mortality per cent.
Immediate end-to-end anastomosis	39	7	17
Closure of ends and lateral anastomosis or implantation	18	3	16
Preliminary colotomy performed or ends brought out after excision	9	3	33

In three cases lateral anastomosis was performed first, and the tumour resected later. In twelve, where the stricture was resected, the subsequent history was traced for a year or more after operation :—

One patient was well 1 year later.
One ,, ,, ,, 1½ years later.
One ,, ,, ,, 2 years later.
One ,, ,, ,, 3 years later.
Two patients were ,, 4 years later.
One patient was ,, 5 years later.
One ,, ,, ,, 7 years later.
One ,, died of general tuberculosis one year after operation.
One ,, ,, tuberculosis several years later.
One ,, ,, phthisis two years, and another three years after operation.

One remained well for three years, then a fistula formed in the operation scar, and in an attempt to close it the patient died.

When the tumour is in the sigmoid flexure, colotomy to relieve the obstruction and give rest to the tumour is certainly the correct treatment; and later, if feasible, it can be excised

Contra-indications to operation are :—

1. Extensive pulmonary tuberculosis, with high temperature.
2. Marked albuminuria.
3. Severe diarrhœa, showing the presence of extensive ulceration.

After operation, the patient should be put under medical treatment and carefully watched to prevent further tuberculous trouble, in the same way as would be done in a case of pulmonary tubercle.

REFERENCES.

F. S. KIDD.—*Lancet*, Jan. 5, 1907.
CROWDER.—*Amer. Jour. Med. Sci.* 1900, 638.
CONRATH.—*Beiträge zur klin. Chir.* 1898, 21.
RECLUS.—*Bull. Méd.* 1893, 587.
PAGE.—*Lancet*, 1897, ii. 10.
LEDIARD.—*Lancet*, 1898, ii. 408.
BERNAY.—*Thèse Lyon*, 1898.
ROLLESTON.—*Trans. Path. Soc.* 1890. xl.

Chapter XV.

CHRONIC CONSTIPATION AND FÆCAL IMPACTION.

CHRONIC CONSTIPATION.

ALTHOUGH it is usual to speak of chronic constipation as a disease, it is nevertheless only a symptom common to a great number of totally distinct and separate affections. Constipation results from the intestinal contents being unduly delayed in their passage along the alimentary canal. This may occur in any part of it, but is most commonly found in the large bowel, and may result from a great variety of causes. It is not possible in these days to consider constipation as a distinct malady, and the first essential always is to ascertain the cause for the condition. Chronic constipation, like many other complaints of the present day, is in most cases a result of modern civilized life. Among native races and wild animals it is practically unknown, but is all too common in civilized communities, and, indeed, forms one of the most frequent disorders of our great cities. Modern methods of dietary and the sedentary character of our daily life are largely responsible for the tendency to constipation which is so prevalent. It is one of the penalties we pay for the comparatively small use we make of our colons.

Dr. Hertz's recent researches, in which patients with severe constipation were examined by the X rays after a bismuth meal, have clearly proved that in most severe chronic cases the delay occurs in the lower part of the colon, and chiefly in the sigmoid flexure. This is the natural receptacle for the fæces previous to dejection. The rectum, being purely an expelling organ, is empty in normal individuals except just previous to and during the act of defæcation. Occasionally, constipation may result from the rectum not acting properly, as in chronic nerve lesions of the spinal cord, but this is comparatively rare.

Being only a symptom, constipation can have no distinctive

CHRONIC CONSTIPATION

pathology, and its causes form a large part of the subject matter of this book, and will be found scattered throughout its pages.

It is obvious that there are two distinct kinds of constipation :

1. That in which the peristaltic power of the colon is normal, but the passage of fæcal material is delayed by the presence of some obstruction in the bowel; and

2. That in which there is no obstruction, but the peristaltic and expulsive power is deficient.

The first is often called obstructive and the second atonic constipation.

There is a third factor, which is often important, though it is not by itself a frequent cause of constipation. This is the consistency of the fæcal material.

The longer fæcal material is delayed in its passage along the colon, the harder will it become, owing to the extraction of water by the bowel walls ; and the harder it becomes the less easily will it be passed along by peristalsis, so that a vicious circle is soon established. The consistency of the fæces, therefore, is often an important factor both in obstructive and atonic constipation. An individual should not be considered as suffering from constipation simply because there is not an action of the bowels daily. Many persons only have such an action three or four times a week, and yet remain in perfect health ; while others again have a normal action twice daily. Constipation is only present when the bowels act with no regularity, or only as the result of aperients.

Constipation is chiefly of importance because of the secondary symptoms to which it gives rise. These symptoms are very numerous, such as headache, dullness, discomfort in the abdomen, backache, furred tongue, etc., but the most important result of severe chronic constipation is the condition often called auto-intoxication. When the contents of the colon are unduly delayed in their passage to the anus, and remain long retained within the body, certain alterations take place. Chemical changes occur in the fæcal material, and many of the waste products of digestion become still further split up into poisonous substances or toxins. Under normal circumstances there would not be time for the formation of poisonous by-products before the fæces are discharged from the body ; but in chronic constipation considerable quantities of these may form while the fæces are still in the colon, and may then be absorbed by the bowel-wall, and find their way into the blood-stream. The patient in fact is slowly poisoned by toxins formed within his own colon.

We have good evidence of the extremely poisonous nature of these toxins in cases of intestinal obstruction. Here, when death occurs, it is more often due to a profound toxæmia from the poisons generated within the obstructed bowel, than from the obstruction itself.

The toxæmia in chronic constipation is never so serious or profound as in intestinal obstruction, because the poisoning occurs more slowly, and the bowel-wall being undamaged, absorption does not occur so readily. It often, nevertheless, produces after a time very serious consequences. The patient becomes lethargic and listless. The appetite is poor, and there is a general feeling of not being well. The skin, instead of looking healthy, becomes of a greyish or earthy colour. The skin smells; the tongue is coated; and frequently much of the subcutaneous fat disappears. There is generally a chronic headache, and sometimes severe neuralgia and even more serious mental symptoms have occurred. The appearance of patients suffering from chronic auto-intoxication is often quite characteristic, the listless appearance and the colour of the skin being alone sufficient to identify them as the subjects of chonic constipation. By no means all sufferers from constipation, however, are the subjects of auto-intoxication. We not infrequently meet with individuals whose bowels act most irregularly and at long intervals, without any apparent ill effects. I have seen at least two patients, whose bowels had not acted for three weeks or a month, who presented no signs of auto-intoxication, and we must assume here either that the poisons are not absorbed or that the patient is immune to their effects.

Atonic constipation results from the muscular action of the bowel-wall being deficient. This is apparently not due to any reduction in the number of the unstriped muscle fibres, but to the absence of the normal stimuli. Peristalsis is normally a reflex action set up by the presence of material within the bowel; in atonic constipation this reflex becomes sluggish. Most often this constipation is a secondary condition resulting from irregular habits in going to stool, improper diet, visceroptosis, or some other general trouble. It may be associated with loss of tone in the abdominal muscles, and this becomes

CHRONIC CONSTIPATION

important, since it is upon these muscles that the expulsion of the fæces chiefly depends.

Among other causes of atonic constipation must be mentioned disease of the central nervous system, such as tabes dorsalis and disseminated sclerosis; neurasthenia is often included, but it seems at least as probable that it is a result.

TREATMENT.

The treatment of chronic constipation obviously depends upon the conditions underlying it, and the correct method is to ascertain these causes and to correct or remove them. When due to obstruction, such as a chronic volvulus, adhesions, a tumour or stricture, operation is clearly indicated. For the treatment of obstructive constipation, the reader is referred to other portions of this book.

In atonic constipation, treatment should be directed to improving the tone of the bowel-wall and increasing the normal stimulus to peristalsis. For this purpose a course of massage, combined, if possible, with suitable electrical treatment, is usually most efficacious if properly carried out. Strychnine or nux vomica are most useful in increasing the peristaltic movements, and their action is often enhanced by the addition of belladonna. At first these drugs should be combined with a small amount of some mild aperient, and later, when they have begun to do good, should be used alone. I have found the following pill most useful in these cases:—

℞
Ext. Colocynth. co.	grs. ix
Ext. Cascaræ	grs. x
Ext. Belladonnæ	grs. iv
Ext. Nucis Vomicæ	grs. iv

Mitte pil. xii.—One or two at bedtime each night.

The results of treatment in cases of chronic constipation are far better where aperients are not used. They are an easy means of getting the bowels to act; but they do not remove the cause of the condition, and, as a rule, ultimately result in making it worse, or in the patient being condemned to continue their use.

Occasionally, where there is a gouty element, the use of some aperient water containing small doses of magnesia and lithia is very beneficial, but with a few exceptions aperients are best avoided.

Enemata are in many cases much to be preferred to the use of aperients, and especially where for long periods some artificial aid has to be used to ensure the bowels acting.

There are frequent instances where the abnormal solidity of the fæces is a most important factor in maintaining the condition; here it will be found that if steps are taken to prevent the fæces from becoming solid a marked improvement will quickly result. In a few cases merely increasing the amount of fluids drunk during the day will be sufficient; but as water is readily absorbed by the colon wall this will only be of service where the patient has been in the habit of taking less fluid than his tissues require, and in whom, therefore, the deficiency has been made up from the fæces.

Fats, which are liquid at body temperature, will prevent the fæces from solidifying, and as only a very limited quantity of fat can be absorbed by the alimentary tract, it is quite easy to attain the desired result by giving an excess of fat in the diet. The addition per diem of two ounces of thick cream to the patient's diet will generally render the stools quite soft, and it is easy to ascertain by experiment the exact quantity of fat required. Salads with oil, milk, bacon, and other forms of diet which contain fat, will readily suggest themselves. Some patients, however, are unable to take an excess of fat without getting dyspepsia.

Mineral fats have not this objection; they are not absorbed at all in their passage through the alimentary canal, but pass out as they went in. Petroleum in some form can be given for any length of time without causing harmful results, and by administering suitable quantities of it any desirable consistency of the fæces can be obtained.

Several different forms of emulsion containing petroleum have recently been placed on the market, and have been much lauded in the treatment of constipation and allied conditions, but emulsions are not so efficacious as pure petroleum, and their only advantage is that they are slightly less greasy to the taste. Lenital is the best preparation, and should be given by the mouth in teaspoonful doses. As a rule a teaspoonful of Lenital three times a day will very quickly render the stools quite soft or even semi-liquid. If not, the

CHRONIC CONSTIPATION

dose should be increased until this result is obtained. It is rather greasy, but otherwise tasteless except for a flavouring of peppermint, and I have found that patients do not object to it or find it unpleasant to take. I have had a number of cases of severe chronic constipation of the atonic type which have entirely recovered by the employment of this simple remedy alone. Even some cases of obstructive constipation are very much improved by rendering the fæces soft, and as an adjunct to massage and electricity it is most useful in cases of constipation due to adhesions. I have had several patients who for years had been in the habit of taking aperients daily, and whose bowels only acted as a result of medicine, who have been able entirely to stop the use of aperients when they began to take petroleum in this form.

MASSAGE.—This is one of the best methods of treating atonic constipation, and cases where there are adhesions interfering with the movements of the bowel. It is also useful after operations undertaken for the cure of obstructive constipation. For the success of this treatment it is essential that a skilled masseur or masseuse be employed; partially trained persons are of little use. Before commencing the massage the patient should be put on a full diet containing plenty of cellulose and a sufficient quantity of fat, or its substitute petroleum, to ensure the fæces being unformed.

If possible, it is better to commence with massage for ten minutes twice a day about two or three hours after meals. This is very much better than one treatment of longer duration, and is more easily borne by the patient. The massage must at first be very gentle, and only slowly increased as the patient becomes accustomed to it. Very vigorous massage is a mistake, and does far less good than light massage. We should aim at moving on the contents of the colon by stimulating peristalsis and by direct kneading of the colon in a direction towards the anus. Special attention should also be paid to the development of the abdominal muscles, and for this purpose the exercises described below are most useful, and may with advantage be combined with the massage. After a few days, if the massage is well borne and does not cause discomfort, each treatment may slowly increased up to twenty minutes twice daily. There is little to be gained by continuing it for more than twenty minutes at one time. As soon as massage is commenced, all aperients should be stopped, if they are being taken. Usually the bowels at once commence to act naturally; should they not do so, enemata of soft soap and water should be used. The massage should be continued daily for at least three weeks, and if possible longer; after this, for two or three times a week for another six weeks or two months. Patients often object to the inconvenience of daily massage; but I have found it most important, unless only temporary benefit is to result from the treatment.

When the patient has sufficiently improved as the result of the treatment, and the bowels are acting regularly, he should be told to take daily exercise, preferably walking or riding; and to make a habit of relieving the bowels at the same time each day. Cannon balls covered with wash-leather, and various forms of rollers, are often used in the treatment of constipation by massage, but if a skilled masseur is obtainable artificial aids are unnecessary.

Vibration, if proper apparatus is used, is also a useful aid to massage in these cases.

EXERCISES FOR DEVELOPING THE ABDOMINAL MUSCLES.—The following exercises should be carried out daily, at first under the supervision of the masseur, and later by the patient for himself. They should be done in succession, and continued about fifteen minutes, but never for long enough to cause fatigue. Each movement should be done slowly and deliberately. When the patient is also having massage, it should follow the exercises.

Exercise 1.—The patient should lie flat on his back on a firm bed or upon the floor, and with his hands by his sides. The knees should be drawn up to the chest, then straightened out at right angles with the trunk. With the knees kept stiff, the legs should then be slowly lowered until they again touch the bed.

Exercise 2.—With the patient lying as before, the right leg, with the knee kept stiff, should be slowly raised till it is at right angles with the body. It should then be slowly lowered again, still with the knee stiff, stopping for a few seconds at different angles with the trunk. Two or three stops should be made before the leg again rests on the bed.

The same exercise should be carried out with the left leg.

Exercise 3.—The patient should lie on the floor with his hands by his sides. Then, while his legs are held down, he should slowly raise himself into a sitting position without using his hands.

The body should then be twisted round, first in one direction and then in the other; he should then slowly lie down again.

Exercise 4.—The patient stands up and slowly raises first one leg and then the other. Each knee should be brought up until it touches the chest.

Exercise 5.—The patient stands with his hands on his hips and slowly rotates the body, first in one direction and then in the other.

Exercise 6.—Repeat Exercise 2, but with both feet together instead of alternately. This and Exercise 7 should not be used at first, but may usefully supplement the foregoing exercises at the end of a week or ten days.

Exercise 7.—The patient sits on the floor, and the feet are held down. He then slowly sways himself backwards and forwards from the hips.

Exercise 8.—(This is to develop the gluteal muscles). With the hands on the hips, the patient squats down on his heels; then slowly raises himself into the standing position, and again slowly lowers himself until he is sitting on his heels. This should be repeated two or three times.

ELECTRICAL TREATMENT.—There are many different kinds of electrical treatment used for chronic constipation; some are quite useless, as they do not cause contraction of the unstriped muscle of the bowel-wall. This especially applies to small galvanic and faradic apparatus which can be obtained for a few pounds; such apparatus are quite valueless for this purpose, and if benefit does occur after their use, it is due to suggestion rather than to electricity.

One of the forms which seems to do most good in atonic cases is the application to the abdomen of a continuous current with quick reversals, one reversal each minute. The pads should be large, and applied one on each side of the abdomen. A cushion must be placed between the knees to prevent their knocking together and becoming bruised. The current should go up to 100 milliampères. Each treatment should last about ten minutes, and not be repeated oftener than thrice a week.

Another very useful form of electricity is the three-phase sinusoidal current. The patient lies on a couch with one large pad in the middle of the back, and two smaller ones, one on each side of the abdomen. The current should not be strong enough to cause any discomfort. The treatment should be continued for about fifteen or twenty minutes, care being taken to switch off the current before putting on or removing the pads, and not to disturb the pads while the current is passing.

The high-frequency current is also useful if properly applied. A good apparatus is essential, and a very high frequency current should be used, with a spark-gap of not less than one and a half inches. The patient should lie on a couch which is not insulated, and should be in good contact with the electrode; that is to say, he should either firmly grasp a metal bar electrode, or have one resting firmly on the abdomen. The administration of the high-frequency current by means of loose and moving contacts, such as brushes or glass electrodes which are moved about, causes pain, and serves, I believe, no good purpose.

The current should always be switched on after the patient is in contact with the electrode, and off before he has released it. If properly administered it should cause no sensation while passing. It should be administered every day for fifteen minutes.

HYDROTHERAPY in its various forms is now very popular for the treatment of chronic constipation, especially at the English and Continental spas. Personally, I have not seen as good results from it as from massage and electricity.

The so-called Plombières treatment, or lavage of the bowel, is not suitable in atonic constipation, as it dilates an already weakened and dilated colon, and, I believe, tends to increase and accentuate the atony of the bowel-wall rather than to improve it. It undoubtedly does temporary good by clearing out the colon and washing away scybala, but the improvement is seldom permanent, while some cases are certainly rendered worse by it. Plombières treatment consists of the daily administration of large enemata, containing a slight quantity of some salt, by means of a long tube. It is supposed that the long tube passes into the colon, but, as I have already pointed out, this is not the case; the tube in most cases remains curled up in the rectum. Any good results obtainable from Plombières treatment can be equally realized by the use of ordinary soap and water enemata when properly administered.

OPERATIVE TREATMENT.—Operations which are performed for chronic constipation without reference to the underlying pathological cause cannot be considered as satisfactory or scientific procedures; before advising operation there should be a clear understanding of the pathological conditions at work, and the manner in which they are to be benefited.

CHRONIC CONSTIPATION

In most cases of obstructive constipation, surgery affords the only satisfactory means of dealing with it or of curing it. The various methods employed will be found elsewhere in this book.

There are certain cases of atonic constipation in which operation is called for; but these are exceptional, and in all of them, if a thorough course of non-operative treatment has not already been tried, it should first be prescribed.

The cases which require operation are those in which the patient is getting seriously ill from auto-intoxication, and the bowels cannot be made to act regularly either by enemata, aperients, or massage. Cases are occasionally met with in which nothing seems to do good, and patient and doctor are in despair. The patient has spent months at spas without any permanent relief; massage only causes discomfort, and only the most drastic aperients, and those in full doses, will relieve the bowels. The patient is always ill, and can think of nothing else but the condition of the bowels, and is rapidly becoming a chronic invalid.

Here an operation is certainly the best treatment, and is quite justified. Three methods have been advised, viz. :—

1. *To perform appendicostomy*, in order that the colon may be washed out daily, and the accumulation of fæcal material within it thereby prevented.

2. *To short-circuit the colon* by performing ileo-sigmoidostomy.

3. *To resect the entire colon*.

Appendicostomy.—It is obvious that it is not the colon which causes auto-intoxication so much as the material which is retained in it. If we can prevent this retention, we shall be able to stop the chronic poisoning from which the patient suffers. If an appendicostomy is performed, the patient is able to wash out the colon daily and so prevent accumulation. The results have in most cases been extremely encouraging, and the daily irrigation has caused rapid and marked improvement in the patient's general condition. Further, in several cases after irrigation has been carried out continuously for some time, there have been signs that the colon was recovering its lost functions, the bowels having begun to act regularly without the irrigation. Appendicostomy has an advantage over the other two operations mentioned, in that it is practically unattended by any risk to life, and that it does not in any way mutilate the patient or leave a condition which may at some later period cause trouble.

Ileo-sigmoidostomy.—In October, 1900, Mr. Mansell Moullin published a case in which he had performed this operation for chronic constipation, and Mr. Arbuthnot Lane published a paper advocating it in 1904.

Mr. Lane, who has performed a number of these operations, found that the results were satisfactory, but that the partially excluded colon was a source of danger, and this has led him to advocate complete resection of the colon as being preferable.

Resection of the Colon.—This has been often performed by Mr. Lane, the ileum being implanted into the rectum or sigmoid flexure.

Frequently a very marked improvement in the patient's general condition resulted from the removal of the colon. The operation is, however, a severe one, and the improvement is not always permanent. Lane has reported 28 cases of excision of the colon for this condition; of these 7 died and 21 recovered. This is a mortality of 33 per cent.

Sufficient time has not yet elapsed to enable us to determine the ultimate results. The mortality in Lane's cases is surprisingly low for so serious an operation; but it seems very doubtful whether a method followed by so high a mortality as 33 per cent is justifiable, especially when appendicostomy seems to be attended with equally good results in similar cases. It is certainly advisable to do appendicostomy first, and only resort to resection if this fails to relieve the symptoms.

FÆCAL IMPACTION.

Occasionally a fæcal mass or enterolith forms in the colon, and causes a condition of chronic, or in a few cases even acute, obstruction. The commonest situation for such fæcal masses is in the rectal ampulla, but they may also be met with in the cæcum, the sigmoid flexure, and at the splenic angle.

Out of the 46 cases collected by Gant, the situation of the calculus or mass was as follows:—

	CASES.
Rectum	35
Sigmoid	5
Descending Colon	1
Transverse Colon	2
Cæcum	3

FÆCAL IMPACTION

They are not infrequently met with in the rectum of old women the subjects of chronic constipation. Under such circumstances they are about the size of an orange and of the consistency of concrete.

Fæcal calculi are most frequently met with in elderly persons, but are not confined to any particular age, and may be found even in children. The concretion is usually single, but cases of multiple calculi have been recorded in which as many as 38 were removed from the same patient.

The composition varies considerably. They may consist of any indigestible material which has been swallowed, such as hair, cotton fibre, and cellulose. The majority, however, are composed of a mixture of inspissated fæces and inorganic salts. The nucleus is generally a foreign body, such as a fruit-stone.

The chemical composition of these stercoliths, apart from the foreign bodies of which they may be composed, is variable ; but the usual ingredients include magnesium and ammonium phosphate, potassium sulphate, sodium carbonate, calcium phosphate, and cholesterin. The centre is usually very hard, and white or colourless. Outside this are concentric layers of earthy matter of varying degrees of hardness.

These calculi are often of considerable size. I have removed one from the rectum which was the size of a child's head.

Fæcal impaction and the formation of enteroliths is never a primary condition ; some abnormality of the colon or rectum, of the nature of obstruction or atony, must necessarily be present. The most distinctive cases of fæcal impaction, in which the mass often weighs several pounds, are those curious instances of congenital dilatation and hypertrophy of the colon. (See *Chap. IV.*).

Fæcal calculi tend to set up inflammation in the surrounding colon, and many of the symptoms they cause are due to this fact. Ulceration, and in a few instances perforation, may occur.

The following rare case, in which a fæcal calculus was found in the splenic flexure, producing obstruction, was recorded by M. Morestin.

Case.—The patient was a woman, aged 31, who had suffered from constipation for two years. Abdominal pains set in during gestation, and a month after delivery a tumour was felt in the abdomen. The patient became ill, with symptoms of chronic obstruction, which were only temporarily relieved by enemata. On opening the abdomen a fæcal calculus of extreme hardness was found in the splenic angle of the colon. This portion of the bowel was resected, together with the calculus, and the colon anastomosed end to end. The patient recovered. The stone required a hammer to break it, and consisted of concentric laminæ. It measured 7 inches in its longest by $5\frac{3}{4}$ inches in its shortest diameter, and weighed 368 grams, about four-fifths of a pound. There was a stricture from old ulceration at the site where the concretion was impacted.

Case.—A case was recorded by M. Pozzi at the French Congress of Surgery in October, 1908, of a man who for years had suffered from an abdominal tumour of absolutely wooden consistency. It extended from the umbilicus to the pelvis, and was movable only in a transverse direction. No exact diagnosis had been made. M. Pozzi performed laparotomy, and found that the tumour consisted of the lower part of the sigmoid flexure, in which was a stercolith of stony hardness. The intestine was divided and the mass removed. The gut was subsequently closed, and the patient made a good recovery.

A similar case is recorded by Balfour Marshall.* :—

Case.—The patient was a woman, aged 46, who complained of a small lump in the abdomen, to which she attributed her symptoms. The chief complaint was of colicky pains. There was a history of constipation. In the lower right quadrant of the abdomen there was a hard ovoid lump, the size of a hen's egg. It was freely movable. It was thought to be either a solid ovarian tumour with a long pedicle, or cancer of the bowel-wall. Laparotomy was performed, and the tumour was found to be a stercolith in the cæcum above a fibrous stricture. The stricture and cæcum were incised and the mass removed. In sewing up the wound in the cæcum the stitches were so inserted as to render the wound transverse instead of longitudinal, thereby increasing the diameter of the strictured area. Recovery was uninterrupted.

Symptoms.

The characteristic symptoms of fæcal calculi are diarrhœa and colic. This not infrequently leads to a wrong diagnosis, as it is sometimes supposed that constipation should result from a fæcal impaction in the colon. The diarrhœa is spurious,

---

* *Glasg. Med. Jour.* 1907, 238.

FÆCAL IMPACTION

and is due to the irritation and ulceration set up by the calculus. If the concretion is in the rectum, tenesmus is a prominent feature. After a time blood and pus may make their appearance in the stools. The stools themselves are thin, watery, and frequent, but small in quantity. The symptoms in fact are those of ulcerative colitis rather than anything else.

In fæcal impaction not due to a calculus, ulceration is less common, and constipation is the rule, accompanied by abdominal colic and sometimes vomiting.

A careful examination both of the rectum and abdomen will generally clear up the diagnosis, as the mass can be felt. If it can be indented the diagnosis is clear, but where a hard calculus is present in some part of the colon where it cannot be seen by the sigmoidoscope, it may be difficult to distinguish the condition from cancer.

Treatment.

When the condition can be diagnosed, attempts should be made to soften the mass by means of large oil enemata, and if this succeeds the mass can be slowly washed out by repeated soap-and-water enemata. A solution of hydrogen peroxide, if it can be brought into contact with a fæcal concretion, will readily split it up and disintegrate it. As the peroxide soaks into the mass, bubbles of gas form in its substance and break it up. While this is a very effective method, it is not free from risk, as the large quantity of gas formed distends the bowel and may rupture it, especially if there is any ulceration. If a free exit for the gas can be ensured, however, this method of breaking up the calculus may be tried.

As a rule, when the calculus is in the colon, surgical operation affords the only possible means of dealing with it. The abdomen should be opened and the portion of the colon containing the calculus brought into the wound. If possible, the calculus should be pressed up into a healthy portion of colon. This should then be incised in the long axis, and the calculus removed. Before closing the incision into the bowel the interior should be examined for a stricture, which is frequently present, and if this is found it should be dealt with at the same time.

It is well to remember that fæcal impaction, or the formation of a calculus, does not occur in a normal colon, and that the presence of one of these conditions indicates some abnormality of the bowel. The following case well exemplifies this statement.

Case.—The patient was an elderly gentleman who for some months had been troubled with constipation, to which he was not accustomed. On examination of the abdomen, his doctor discovered a tumour in the left iliac fossa, and asked me to see the patient with a view to ascertaining its nature. Before I saw him a dose of castor oil and several enemata had been administered, and as a result the tumour had disappeared. An attempt to examine him with the sigmoidoscope failed, as the bowel was still loaded with fæces. We came to the conclusion that the tumour had been a fæcal mass, but that a further examination after the bowel had been emptied was advisable to ascertain the cause of the accumulation. To this, however, he would not agree, as he considered himself cured. A year later this patient had an attack of acute obstruction, and colotomy was performed. It was then discovered that there was a cancer of the sigmoid flexure, which had doubtless been present before, and could have been detected had he submitted to be examined properly.

Chapter XVI.

SIMPLE STRICTURE OF THE COLON AND EMBOLISM OF THE MESOCOLIC VESSELS.

SIMPLE STRICTURE.

COMPARED with malignant stricture this is a rare condition. Cases of simple (non-malignant) stricture may be divided into three kinds :—

1. Stricture due to hyperplastic tuberculosis.
2. Stricture due to pericolitis.
3. Cicatricial strictures the result of ulceration.

The first two conditions are commonly mistaken for cancer, and so close is the resemblance that it is often only possible to be certain of their benign nature after careful microscopical examination. Both in hyperplastic tuberculosis and pericolitis the stricture is accompanied by considerable tumour formation. These conditions will, however, not be further considered here, as they have already been described in Chapters XIII. and XIV.

Cicatricial stricture of the colon is a very rare condition. Out of 669 cases of intestinal obstruction collected by the late H. L. Barnard from the records of the London Hospital, there were only four of simple stricture of the colon, and these were all in the sigmoid flexure.

Simple stricture of the colon, as also of the rectum, has been supposed to be a result of tertiary syphilis ; but after careful search, I have not succeeded in finding a single instance of an undoubted syphilitic lesion, much less of a syphilitic stricture.

It may be congenital, and in Chapter VI. several such cases are given. The commonest cause is undoubtedly the contraction following severe chronic ulceration. As I have already pointed out, most ulcers of the colon heal, if at all, without leaving much scarring. If the ulcer is very large, however, and has entirely destroyed the mucous membrane, scarring and contraction may result. This is especially the case with chronic ulcers.*

I have seen one case of a diaphragm-like stricture of the pelvic colon in which the condition appeared to have resulted from previous ulceration. In St. Bartholomew's Hospital museum there is a very interesting specimen (see *Fig.* 58) of a cicatricial stricture in the middle of the transverse colon. There are a number of curious thread-like polypi hanging from the mucous membrane in the neighbourhood of the stricture. Curiously enough, dysenteric ulceration apparently never results in stricture. Thus, out of the records of 287,522 cases of dysentery occurring among the troops in the American Civil War, there was no single instance of a stricture of the colon.

A very moderate degree of stricture in the descending or pelvic portions of the colon will cause obstruction, owing to the solid nature of the contents. When acute obstruction occurs from a simple stricture, the actual cause of the blockage is always fæcal impaction.

Most of these cicatricial strictures are complicated by the presence of adhesions around the bowel which, like the stricture, have resulted from the previous ulceration.

The changes which occur in the bowel above the stricture are those usually associated with a chronic partial obstruction. The bowel is dilated and its walls are markedly hypertrophied. Stercoral ulceration may be present, and in some cases multiple polypi have been found growing from the mucous membrane just above the stricture. The formation of stercoliths thus situated has already been referred to in Chapter XV.

TREATMENT.

The condition may be treated either by resection of the affected

---

* The following case is recorded by Quénu and Duval (*Rev. de Chirurgie*, Dec. 10, 1902). The patient was a man, age 67. For some time he had complained of pain in the abdomen, and suffered from habitual constipation. His bowels were for long periods unrelieved. Examination of the abdomen revealed a hard cylindrical mass in the cæcal region. Nothing could be felt per rectum, and intestinal obstruction probably due to cancer was diagnosed. The patient refused to be operated upon, and died. Post mortem, a large abscess cavity, shut off by adhesions, was discovered in the lower part of the abdomen. This cavity communicated with the sigmoid flexure by a perforation at the bottom of an old ulcer. The contraction of the ulcer had caused an annular constriction which almost occluded the bowel.

portion of bowel, or by incising the bowel-wall over and through the stricture, and then sewing up the resulting wound in a transverse direction. The operation is, however, often much complicated by the presence of adhesions in the neighbourhood, and it may sometimes be better to deal with the case by short-circuiting the affected portion of bowel by lateral anastamosis.

THROMBOSIS OR EMBOLISM OF THE COLIC BLOOD-VESSELS.

Embolism of one of the main arteries of the colon, or thrombosis of the veins, results in complete obstruction. The contents of the colon are arrested and the bowel above becomes distended. Thrombosis is a very rare condition, and is but seldom diagnosed during life.

The symptoms produced by embolism or thrombosis are those of intestinal obstruction, and it is not possible to make a correct diagnosis unless there is some reason to expect embolism. Exactly why an infarcted portion of the colon should produce obstruction it is not easy to see ; but it apparently acts as a complete block to the passage of the intestinal contents, and the bowel above becomes dilated as if a stricture were present. When seen, the appearance of the bowel is characteristic. It is of a dark chocolate colour, and in marked contrast to the surrounding healthy bowel. When laid open, the mucous membrane is seen to be purplish in colour and œdematous.

For the notes of the following case, which well illustrate this rare and interesting condition, I am indebted to Mr. Littlewood, of Leeds.

The patient was a woman, aged 64. She was much wasted. There was a history of several days' complete intestinal obstruction, with fæcal vomiting and some abdominal distention. There was no history of melæna, and no evidence on examination of any cardiac lesion.

An exploratory laparotomy was performed. The patient was very ill, and died on the operating-table. A post-mortem examination revealed in the left half of the transverse colon a portion about $2\frac{1}{2}$ to 3 inches in length which was thickened and œdematous. The corresponding portion of mesocolon was similarly thickened, and both this and the bowel-wall were markedly injected. On opening the gut, the mucous membrane was seen to be of a chocolate colour, and slightly swollen. The affected portion of mucous membrane was, owing to the change in colour, sharply marked off from the normal mucosa. There was well-marked venous dilatation.

Thrombosis was discovered. One small artery near the bowel contained blood-clot, but the clot was not apparently attached to the vessel wall. The colon was distended, and the discoloured portion of the transverse colon marked the junction between the distended and collapsed portions of bowel. The cæcum was greatly distended, and there was distention of the ascending and right half of the transverse colon; but the distention terminated at the discoloured portion of bowel, and the descending colon was collapsed.

The remainder of the intestine was quite normal, as were also the other abdominal organs.

Treatment.

When an extensive area of colon is involved, it is unlikely that any operative or other treatment will avail. But if the infarcted area is not large, and operation is performed early, resection of the whole damaged area of bowel will probably save the patient's life.

It is unlikely that the condition will be diagnosed previous to operation; but as the symptoms are those of intestinal obstruction, a condition calling for immediate operative interference, this is not a serious obstacle to a successful result.

Chapter XVII.

SIMPLE TUMOURS OF THE COLON.

SIMPLE tumours are not very common in the colon. Fibrous tumours, the result of diverticula and pericolitis, and hyperplastic tuberculosis, are sometimes found, and have already been referred to under these headings. These fibrous tumours, however, are inflammatory in origin, and not true tumours. Lipomata are occasionally found in connection with the colon; but they are rare, and seldom cause symptoms unless of very large size. Mr. Bland-Sutton, in his book on tumours, relates a case in which he removed a lipoma of the ascending colon which was causing obstruction.

Villous adenomata occur in the colon; but they are seldom detected before they have become malignant. In most cases, when removed, they are found to show well-marked malignant changes, and are therefore usually classified as malignant tumours. Single polypi are occasionally met with, and are a well-known cause of intussusception; their structure is usually adenomatous, and they have a long pedicle produced by the action of peristalsis in attempting to move them along the bowel lumen.

Multiple Polypi of the Colon.—One of the most interesting and curious forms of simple tumour of the colon is the condition described as multiple polypi. It is also described as multiple adenomata and colitis polyposa.

The condition is rare; but I have been able to collect a number of cases; and several drawings and photographs of the condition are appended.

"Multiple polypi of the colon" is not a pathological entity, but includes several distinct diseases which have been described under this name.

Multiple polypi may be divided into four classes, as follows :—(1) *True multiple adenomata;* (2) *Polypi found in association with hyperplastic tuberculosis;* (3) *Multiple polypi found in association with an old stricture of the colon;* (4) *The polypoid condition of the mucosa which sometimes results from ulcerative colitis.*

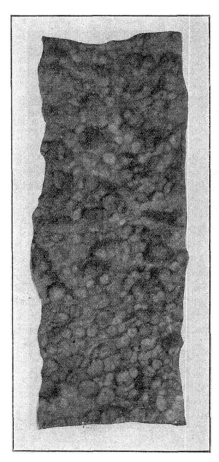

Fig. 53.—Multiple adenomata. (*Mr. Fredb. Wallis's case.* Charing Cross Hospital Museum.)

1. **True Multiple Adenomata.**—This is a curious condition in which there are numbers of small adenomata growing from the mucous membrane of the colon. It was first described by Virchow in a paper written in 1863.

OF THE COLON

The number and size of the polypi vary considerably in different cases. They may be quite small and very numerous, so numerous in fact that the entire colon is covered with them, or they may be large and comparatively limited in number.

There appear to be two distinct types : one in which the entire colon is covered with small semi-pedunculated polyps in such

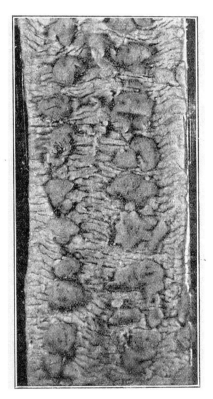

Fig. 54.—Multiple polypi of the colon (Charing Cross Hospital Museum).

numbers that the mucosa is almost hidden. The two best-marked cases of this type are :—Mr. F. Wallis's case, the specimen of which is in Charing Cross Hospital (see *Fig.* 53), and Lienthall's case. In the former there was a similar condition in the stomach, and in part of the small intestine, and the condition

240 SIMPLE TUMOURS

resembled lymphadenoma. In Lienthall's case the disease was apparently confined to the colon. This type is extremely rare.

In the other and commoner class there are numerous polypi of all sizes and shapes, some of them sessile, but the majority pedunculated. The sessile polypi appear to be but the early condition of the large pedunculated ones. They are often large, and may have pedicles an inch or more in length. In one

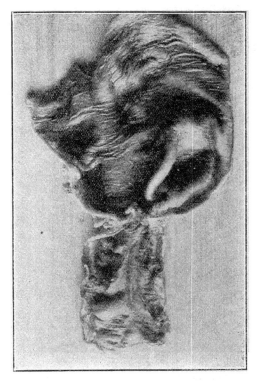

Fig. 55.—Multiple polypi of the colon, associated with a cancerous stricture.
(From a specimen in the Great Northern Hospital Museum.)

of my cases a polypus which broke off and was passed per anum was as large as a walnut, and had a long narrow, ribbon-like stem.

There may be great numbers of these polypi distributed

throughout the colon. There are usually numerous quite small and undeveloped polypi to be seen, and if these are examined they are found to be growing from the free edges of the valvulæ conniventes. An examination of several specimens makes it seem probable that the polypi all originate as outgrowths from the edges of these folds. (See *Fig.* 57.)

They are, as a rule, most numerous in the pelvic and descending portions of the colon. The rectum is also commonly affected. The polypi in the rectum are naturally the most easily detected, and in several instances the condition is described as multiple polypi of the rectum. But I have found no case in which the condition was confined to the rectum; careful investigation or post-mortem examination always proves the colon also to be affected, while in some the rectum is not affected at all.

The condition is always accompanied by a certain amount of inflammation of the mucous membrane, and gives rise to severe and intractable diarrhœa and hæmorrhage.

THE MICROSCOPICAL APPEARANCES. — When sections are examined under the microscope these polypi can be seen to consist of a central mass of typical adenoid tissue, covered outside with the ordinary columnar-celled epithelium of the colon. They are not, however, simple outgrowths or excrescences of the mucous membrane, as the submucous coat is represented. A careful microscopical examination shows that they originate beneath the mucous membrane, probably in the solitary follicles, and, as they protrude into the bowel, become covered and surrounded by the mucous membrane. In the pedunculated variety there is, as a rule, no adenoid tissue in the pedicle, which consists of a tube of mucous membrane enclosing connective tissue continuous with the submucous layer of the bowel-wall.

Little is known as to the etiology of these polypi. The condition occurs at all ages and about equally in the two sexes. The most probable explanation is that they arise from irritation. I recently saw a case in which the condition occurred in a child of four as the result of worms. The fact, already mentioned, that there are almost invariably chronic inflammatory changes in the mucous membrane, supports the same view, which is further strengthened by polypi being often found associated with simple stricture of the colon and with hyperplastic tuberculosis.

SECONDARY CHANGES IN THE POLYPI.—The larger polypi,

SIMPLE TUMOURS

especially those near the lower end of the pelvic colon, tend to become ulcerated from the traumatism to which they are subjected by the passage of the fæces.

What is of much greater importance, however, is, that there is a marked tendency for some of the polypi to become malignant and cause an adeno-carcinomatous stricture. This is particularly liable to occur at those parts of the colon, such as the sigmoid

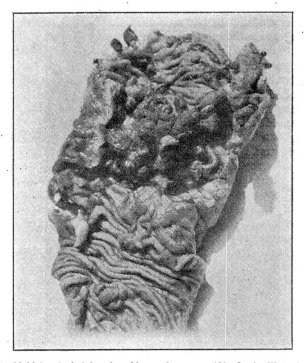

Fig. 56.—Multiple polypi of the colon with secondary cancer (*Mr. Gordon Watson's case*).

flexure, where the polypi are most numerous and most subjected to traumatism from hard fæcal material.

In two of my cases there was already a cancerous stricture in the sigmoid flexure ; and in another there was evidence of cancer some months after the case was first seen. In this latter case numerous polypi could be seen with the sigmoidoscope in the sigmoid flexure and the rectum. All the polypi in the rectum that could be reached were removed. One of these was examined, and showed the typical structure of simple adenoma. Some months later the patient developed symptoms of cancer in the sigmoid, but was too ill to return to the hospital.

In one of the cases there was a carcinomatous stricture in the sigmoid, which was resected. On examination of the specimen it was evident that the growth had arisen in one of the polypi. Two of the polypi at some distance from the growth were examined, and while one was a simple adenoma, the other showed signs of commencing malignancy. (See *Fig.* 56.)

Out of the forty-two cases of multiple polypi of the rectum or colon collected by Quénu and Landel, in twenty cancer was either present when the case was examined, or developed later.

In one of my cases the patient was operated upon for cancer of the sigmoid, and the bowel was resected. No polypi were seen in the resected portion ; but a year later he returned with recurrence of symptoms, and on examination with the sigmoidoscope several pedunculated polypi were seen, some six inches above the old line of anastomosis. The patient died from a second operation, and, post mortem, there were some half-dozen polypi, the highest of which was eight inches above the line of the original anastomosis. There was no recurrence at the original site ; but on examining several of the polypi, two were found to be malignant.

Symptoms.

The most marked symptom is diarrhœa. This is severe and intractable. The patient rapidly wastes and becomes emaciated as the result of the constant loss of fluid, and there is not infrequently considerable tenesmus. The stools are liquid and contain much slimy mucus. Blood is frequently present in the stools and is intimately mixed with them. The symptoms closely resemble those of cancer or ulceration of the colon ; but the diarrhœa is, as a rule, more severe. Abdominal pain is usually present, and in most of the cases there has been severe pain in the left side of the abdomen. There is, as stated before, often marked anæmia.

There is usually a history of bleeding and diarrhœa for long periods. Thus, in one patient there had been almost continuous bleeding for ten years ; and in another the symptoms had persisted without intermission for three. In one very remarkable instance three members of a family suffered from the condition; but I have been unable to find another similar case.

An examination of the rectum usually reveals the presence of a number of polypi scattered over the mucous membrane, and the sigmoidoscope shows a similar condition in the pelvic colon. The colon is tender when palpated through the abdominal wall.

The following are typical cases of the condition :—

Author's Case.—A woman, aged 57. The patient was quite well until August, 1907, when she began to suffer from diarrhœa. This continued intermittently until October, when she began to notice blood in the stools, and had severe pain in the left side of the abdomen. These symptoms continued until her admission to hospital in January, 1908. At this time there were constant diarrhœa and much blood and mucus in the stools. On examination, there were numerous polypi in the rectum. The sigmoidoscope showed numerous polypi growing from the mucous membrane of the pelvic colon as far up as could be seen. They varied in size from quite small sessile polyps to pedunculated growths nearly as large as a walnut. At one spot there was some ulceration of one of the polyps, which suggested possible commencing malignant disease. Under an anæsthetic some of the polypi in the rectum were removed, and on examination showed a simple adenomatous structure. The patient left the hospital and returned home. When heard from in November she was still very ill, and there appeared to be symptoms of malignant stricture. In December her doctor sent me a large polypus which had passed per anum; on having sections of it cut, the typical structure of an adeno-carcinoma could be seen, so that there was no doubt malignant change had occurred.

Case of Multiple Polypi of the Colon Associated with Cancerous Stricture of the Sigmoid Flexure.—Specimen in St. Bartholomew's Hospital Museum (No. 2065). The patient was a man, aged 20, who died in the hospital. Ten years previously he was taken into the London Hospital for hæmorrhage from the bowel, and was operated upon there. The bleeding returned in a few months; and, at intervals, he had hæmorrhage for the next four years. Several further operations were performed, and polypi removed; but with only temporary relief from the bleeding. A brother and sister of this patient were also under treatment at St. Bartholomew's, and were found on examination

OF THE COLON

also to have multiple polypi of the bowel. On admission the patient was very anæmic, and complained of pain in the rectum. There was an almost constant discharge of blood and mucus from the bowel. On dilating his rectum under an anæsthetic numerous polypi could be seen in the rectum, and several of these were removed. He was re-admitted into the hospital

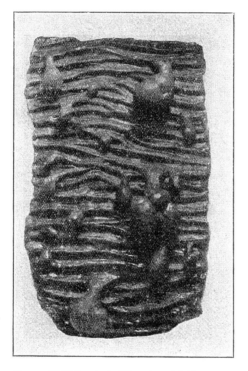

Fig. 57.—Multiple polypi of the colon. (*Author's case.*)

three times, on the last occasion with symptoms of peritonitis, from which he died.

An examination of the specimen shows an adeno-carcinomatous growth at the recto-sigmoidal junction surrounding the bowel and almost obliterating it. Below the stricture there are numerous polypoid growths scattered over the bowel walls. There are also several above the stricture, and in the ascending and transverse portions of the colon are three or four polypi. The colon above the stricture is enormously dilated, and the peritoneum over the anterior band has split from the distention. Most of the polypi are globular, with narrow pedicles, but some are sessile or ribbon-like structures. The microscopical examination shows the growth to be an adeno-carcinoma. The polypi are simple adenomata.

A case* is reported by A. Samuels of a woman, aged 48, who for three-and-a-half years had suffered from frequent watery stools containing blood, and occasional vomiting. There was constant pain in the left side and considerable loss of weight. The abdomen was opened and the colon incised. Numerous polypi were found in the colon, and a large number were removed. The patient was better after operation; but there were occasional recurrences during the next two years. Microscopically the polypi removed proved to be simple adenomata.

2. **Polypi in Association with Hyperplastic Tuberculosis.**—These have already been described in dealing with tubercle of the colon. They occur in or just above the stricture. They may contain giant cells and tubercle bacilli. They may be present in considerable numbers and have long pedicles.

3. **Polypi in Association with an old Stricture.**—These polypi are very curious. They are filiform structures, often of most curious and eccentric shapes, and several inches long. They are often looped or fork-shaped. They are in appearance quite unlike the polypi previously described; and are only found in and just above and below an old simple stricture. (See *Fig.* 58.) They consist of connective tissue covered by mucous membrane.

4. **Polypoid Condition Associated with Ulcerative Colitis.**—These are not true polypi, though their appearance is very similar, but are the islands of mucous membrane left between the ulcerated areas. Each of these becomes partly undermined by the ulceration, and thus a pedicle is formed. The mucous membrane becomes swollen and hypertrophied, and in this way the appearance of a polypus is produced.

TREATMENT OF CASES OF MULTIPLE POLYPI OF THE COLON.

Those forms of polypi accompanying tuberculosis and stricture

---

* *Surg. Gynæcol. and Obstet.* 1909, p. 380.

OF THE COLON

of the colon do not call for any treatment apart from the condition with which they are associated.

The treatment of multiple adenomata is a very difficult matter. In most cases the condition has only been detected in the rectum, and it has been supposed that the polypi were confined to this part of the bowel, whereas they really extended more or less throughout the large bowel. Most of the operations

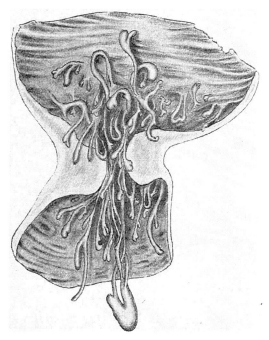

Fig. 38.—Drawing of a specimen in St. Bartholomew's Hospital Museum, showing a simple fibrous stricture in the centre of the transverse colon, and numerous filiform polypi growing from the mucous membrane above the stricture. The colon above the stricture is dilated.

performed have been confined to the removal of as many polypi as possible from the rectum, and in some cases forty or fifty have thus been removed. Such operations have, however, done no good, and the symptoms have persisted as before. In a few the anus and rectum have been laid open, to enable more polypi to be reached. Left inguinal colotomy has also been done with the object of deflecting the fæcal current ; but has been equally useless, because the opening was not above the disease.

Cæcostomy has also been performed. This was done in Lienthall's case, and the patient's symptoms were somewhat alleviated ; but no diminution in the size or number of the polypi resulted.

None of these operations seem of the least use, and they should certainly not be performed. Colotomy does not relieve the symptoms, and merely adds to the patient's distress.

The disease is a very serious one. The patient suffers from severe and intractable diarrhœa and bleeding. There is often severe and distressing tenesmus, and rapid loss of weight and wasting. Moreover, there is every probability that cancer will develop, if it has not already done so.

Under these circumstances any operation would seem justifiable that affords a possibility of removing the disease. The only method that offers any reasonable prospect of dealing adequately with it is resection of the entire colon. This was done in Lienthall's case after a previous ileo-sigmoidostomy, and the patient recovered. This was probably the first instance in which resection of the entire colon was performed.

Unfortunately, the rectum is usually affected together with the colon, so that the whole of the disease cannot be removed ; but if the anastomosis is made low down, the polypi in the rectum could in most cases be removed later ; and, at any rate, this operation seems to be the only one at all worth considering.

Resection of a cancer of the colon which is found to be associated with multiple polypi is apparently not worth doing unless the rest of the colon is either removed at the same time or subsequently. The evidence available seems to show that cancer will recur in some other part of the colon if it has not already done so.

Chapter XVIII.

MALIGNANT DISEASE OF THE COLON.

The commonest form of malignant disease met with in the colon is adeno-carcinoma. Cancer of the colon is a comparatively common disease; indeed, of all the different diseases to which the colon is liable, cancer is probably one of the commonest. Neither is it confined to the later periods of life, for it appears often to affect the colon at an earlier age than with many other parts of the body. Out of 100 cases collected from various sources, I found that eleven were under 30 years of age, and four under 20. The youngest patient was a child, age 5, and another was only 12 years old. Mr. Mayo Robson also records the case of a child aged 14 with cancer of the colon.

The two sexes seem to be about equally affected. In my series 55 patients were males and 45 females.

SITUATION OF THE GROWTH.—The following four series of cases show the comparative frequency of cancer in different portions of the colon :—

Situation	London Hospital.	Clogg's Series.	Tuttle's Series.	Lichtenstein's Series.
Cæcum	41	17	} 283	32
Ascending Colon	6	—		6
Hepatic Flexure	3	5		} 30
Transverse Colon	17	3		
Splenic Flexure	12	10	160	
Descending Colon	6	—		11
Sigmoid Flexure	103	37	182	42
Total	188	72	625	121

It will thus be seen that the sigmoid flexure is the commonest situation; next the cæcum and ascending colon; then the transverse colon or splenic flexure. The parts least commonly affected are the hepatic flexure and the descending colon. The dependent parts of the colon are those most commonly affected with cancer, namely the cæcum, middle of the transverse colon, and the sigmoid flexure. It is in these regions of the bowel that stagnation of the contents tends to occur most frequently.

PREDISPOSING CAUSES OF CANCER OF THE COLON.—Of the real causes of cancer of the colon, or elsewhere, we at present know nothing, and the predisposing causes are chiefly of importance in that they may help us in forming an opinion as to the prognosis in cases in which we know that such causes exist, and in determining whether or no an operation should be undertaken to remove some lesion which may later become a site of cancer. Prof. Nothnagel has stated that cancer of the bowel not infrequently arises at the site of an ulcer of simple origin in the mucous membrane.

That a congenital abnormality of the colon may be a predisposing cause seems probable. A case is recorded by Lockwood, in which the descending colon was double, and at the site of junction of the two tubes there was a cancerous tumour.

Polypi appear to be a common predisposing cause of cancer. The history in many cases clearly shows their presence for a considerable time before the cancer started. These cases are dealt with in full in considering the subject of multiple polypi.

MORBID ANATOMY.—Cancer of the colon always originates in the glands of Lieberkühn, and is of the so-called columnar-celled variety, or aden-ocarcinoma. No other type of carcinoma occurs in the colon, though there may be considerable variations due to secondary or degenerative changes. Colloid degeneration is not uncommon, and in rapidly growing tumours the so-called encephaloid type of degeneration is seen. Occasionally there is a tendency for the fibrous-tissue elements to preponderate, and this results in the scirrhous type of growth. Scirrhous carcinoma is most common in growths of the sigmoid; but it is always a rare form of cancer of the colon. The scirrhous growths do not project into the bowel, but cause a tight stricture of the lumen due to the growth spreading circularly in the submucous layer. The appearance of such tumours is often that of a tight ring-like stricture, the outside of the bowel being grooved as if a string had been tied round it. These scirrhous growths may cause considerable stricture without any ulceration of the mucosa.

The common adeno-carcinoma is a more or less nodular or cauliflower-like outgrowth of the mucosa projecting into the

PLATE V

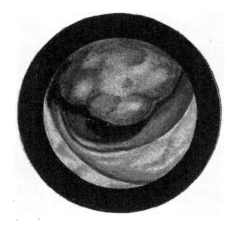

Cancer of the Pelvic Colon as seen through the sigmoidoscope.

bowel lumen. The surface may or may not be ulcerated, depending upon the time it has existed and the amount of traumatism to which it has been subjected. On the outside of the bowel, over the base of such a tumour, there is generally a scar-like depression or hollow, and in addition to the narrowing of the lumen caused by the tumour, there is almost invariably a certain amount of contraction. Rarely, the tumour exists as a polypus hanging loose in the bowel lumen, and in one of my cases there were several such polypi showing malignant changes. (See *Fig. 64*.)

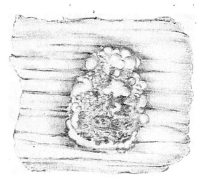

Fig. 59.—An early carcinomatous ulcer of the sigmoid flexure. Resected by the author from a man, age 46.

All cancers found in the colon are, however, essentially the same, namely, adeno-carcinomata, and the various different types often described are merely due to degenerative or other changes.

Cancer of the colon is almost invariably a primary lesion; but there are a few rare and interesting cases where the growth appears to be secondary to another, higher up in the alimentary canal. In these rare instances of secondary carcinoma the infection appears to have been direct. That is, the cancer cells from one growth have apparently passed down the bowel and become implanted in the mucous membrane of the colon, presumably through an abrasion or some breach of surface. It is, of course, possible that the two growths have arisen separately, and have no connection with each other; but in at least one of the cases the appearances suggested that the lower growth was secondary to the upper one.

In a case recorded by Mr. C. Morton,* the cæcum was excised for cancer, and the ileum anastomosed to the ascending colon. The patient recovered ; but five years later there was a cancer in the transverse colon, and the patient died after an operation for its removal.

I have found several instances of more than one growth in the same colon in different parts.

Mr. Littlewood recently reported two such cases.† In one, the patient, a woman aged 52, had a cancer in the splenic flexure of the colon, and another in the rectum. In the other case, a man aged 69 had a cancer in the ascending colon and another similar growth in the rectum.

A case of particular interest is recorded by Mr. G. Simpson,‡ in which there were two primary growths in the colon. One was in the cæcum ; and on microscopical examination was found to be a columnar-celled growth undergoing colloid degeneration ; and the other was in the hepatic flexure, and was a typical scirrhous cancer with numbers of irregular cells arranged in lines.

Metastatic growths of the colon secondary to cancer in parts of the body other than the alimentary tract are very uncommon. Such a case is, however, recorded by Mr. Arbuthnot Lane. The patient was a woman, who many years previously had had her breast removed for cancer. There were no signs of recurrence in the scar or glands, but a growth in the sigmoid was detected. At the operation a cancerous growth was found extending from the mesentery into the sigmoid and stricturing it. Other growths were found of a similar nature in the rectum and in the ascending colon. There was also growth in the liver. The whole colon was removed and the ileum stitched into the anus. The patient died three weeks later. It was found that the growths were secondary carcinoma, and involved in a varying degree almost the whole colon.

The following remarkable case of several separate malignant growths in the colon was under my care at St. Mark's Hospital :

Case.—The patient, a man aged 46, had a small adeno-carcinoma in the centre of his sigmoid flexure. This was successfully resected, and he remained apparently well for nine months, when he was examined

---

* *Brit. Med. Jour.*, Oct. 29, 1904.   † *Lancet*, Jan. 11, 1907.
‡ *Brit. Med. Jour.* Dec. 7, 1907.

with the sigmoidoscope because he was again passing blood. It was then seen that he had several large polypi, some six inches or more above the line of the previous resection, the intervening mucous membrane being normal. One of these polypi was removed, and on examination was found to be a typical carcinoma. A second operation was performed, but the patient died from peritonitis. Post mortem, six of these polypi with long slender stalks were discovered, the highest of which was nine inches above the growth originally removed. Two of these were examined, and one showed typical cancer formation. There were no signs of secondary deposits anywhere. The only reasonable explanation of this curious case seems to be that the original growth resulted from a simple polypus which had become malignant, and that, later, the remaining polypi also took on malignant change.

THE LINES OF EXTENSION OF THE GROWTH.—The study of the directions and ways in which cancer of the colon extends is of the utmost importance, for unless these are known it is not possible to so plan an operation as to be reasonably certain of removing the entire growth. And it is only when operations for cancer are planned according to the known methods of extension of the growth that really successful results can be obtained.

As already stated, cancer when it affects the colon tends for a long time to remain localized to the bowel-wall, and it is exceptional to find the glands in the mesocolon, and especially the retro-peritoneal glands, involved, except in very late cases. Out of thirty cases in which glands were specially looked for, enlarged glands were present in the mesocolon in only five, and retro-peritoneal glands in only three cases. In only two cases was there a secondary deposit in the liver. The thirty were all cases in which an operation had been performed, and not those reaching the post-mortem table after dying from cancer. Of course, a much higher proportion of secondary deposits would be found if cases of advanced and inoperable disease were taken.

At the stage when cancer of the colon is usually detected, enlargement of the glands in the root of the mesocolon and behind the posterior peritoneum is exceptional, the growth tending rather to spread in the bowel-wall, and to involve only those glands in immediate contact with it. We are too apt to assume, because enlarged glands are found in the neighbourhood of a malignant growth, that they are therefore the seat of cancer cells. Frequently, however, this is not the case.

Mr. Clogg, in a similar investigation, found that in only two-thirds of the cases in which there were enlarged glands could cancer cells be found.

While enlarged glands are not uncommonly present in immediate proximity to the growth, and in the fat around the bowel, they are not very common at the root of the mesocolon

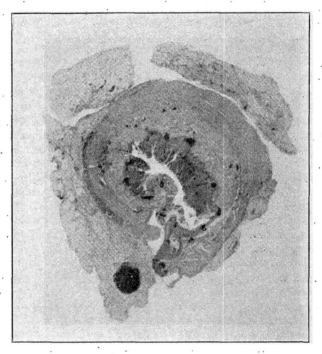

Fig. 60.—Cancer of the sigmoid flexure. A transverse microscopical section of the colon through the centre of the growth. The gland in the lower edge does not show any cancer cells. The growth is spreading in the submucous layer. Photograph from a specimen prepared by Mr. Lenthal Cheatle.

or in the retro-peritoneal tissue; and in many cases the glands that are enlarged are not cancerous. While there are certainly exceptions, as a rule cancer of the colon grows very slowly, and seldom gives rise to secondary deposits in glands or other viscera. I have seen a patient who six years previously had colotomy performed for cancer at the recto-sigmoidal junction (a piece of the growth was at that time removed and examined microscopically), and who was still in good health and free from any signs of secondary deposits. Mr. Swinford Edwards had a similar case, in which the patient lived for over five years without secondary deposits forming. When secondary deposits do occur, they are invariably found in the liver, and practically never elsewhere unless they are also present in the liver.

Invasion of other organs, such as the stomach, bladder, and small intestine, are not uncommon, but these do not come under the head of secondary deposits.

Though cancer of the colon does not, as a rule, spread rapidly, and but seldom causes secondary deposits, its victims do not often live long, as it soon produces obstruction, and, if unoperated upon, a quite small and localized growth will bring about a fatal result in a very few months..

Cancer of the Ileocæcal Angle.—This is, next to the sigmoid flexure, the commonest situation for cancer of the colon. The commonest situation for the growth to start is at the ileocæcal valve; other situations being on the posterior cæcal wall, at the junction of the cæcum and ascending colon, and in the appendix.

Cancer of the Transverse Colon.—Growths in this situation tend very soon to involve the stomach. Out of eight cases of cancer of the transverse colon of which I have notes, four had spread to the stomach, and in two a fistula communicated between the colon and stomach.

Cancer of the Sigmoid Flexure.—This may occur in any part of the sigmoid flexure; but the commonest situations are at about its centre,—that is to say, at the apex of the loop and at the recto-sigmoidal junction.

Symptoms.

These are most variable, and depend upon a number of factors, such as the type and stage of the disease, the situation, and the condition of the patient. So greatly do the symptoms vary in different cases, that we might almost say that any symptom referable to the colon may be produced by cancer.

None, unfortunately, are characteristic. As a rule, they are at first those of an irritative lesion in the colon, and later of a stenosis. A growth may exist in the colon for long periods without producing any symptoms of importance,

MALIGNANT DISEASE

or causing the patient any serious inconvenience. Often the earliest sign is some irregularity in the action of the bowels. There may be slight attacks of diarrhœa, occurring fairly frequently and without any apparent cause ; or, on the other hand,

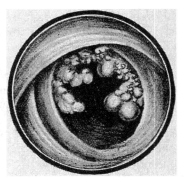

Fig. 61.—Tumour high up in the sigmoid flexure (sigmoidoscopic).

the bowels, which had previously been regular, have a tendency to become constipated, and occasional aperients are required. Sometimes again, the first symptom is the presence of mucus in the stools, either as slime or casts, and accompanied by slight

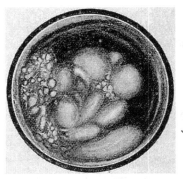

Fig. 62.—Malignant growth at the lower end of the sigmoid flexure growing from the anterior bowel-wall (sigmoidoscopic).

diarrhœa. Such cases are usually first diagnosed as chronic colitis ; and I have seen seven such cases which proved on examination to be cancer of the pelvic colon. Pain or discomfort in the abdomen is often an early symptom. The pain may either take the form of occasional attacks of colic, or of a more or less constant sense of abdominal discomfort, often described as a dull, dragging pain. Flatulence, requiring the constant passage of wind, is another early symptom in some cases.

I recently saw a patient who complained of slight colicky pain coming on in the afternoon after he had been standing for some time, and the presence of mucus in the stools. These symptoms had begun about nine months previously as the result of an attack of indigestion. There were no other symptoms, and the patient looked in excellent health; but a sigmoidoscopic examination revealed a cancerous ulcer in the sigmoid flexure. I once saw a case in which the first symptom of a growth in the sigmoid flexure was a sudden and severe hæmorrhage from the rectum; but this is unusual. As a rule, bleeding is conspicuous by its absence in the early stages of cancer of the colon. The onset of symptoms is often quite abrupt, and may be attributed by the patient to some dietary indiscretion.

It is obvious that the symptoms just detailed are so comparatively insignificant, and so common as the result of other and less important conditions, that it is improbable they should give rise to any suspicion of cancer of the colon. Certainly no one would venture to make a diagnosis of growth upon such evidence. Nevertheless, they are of the utmost importance, for if we are to treat cancer of the colon successfully, we must be able to diagnose the condition while the growth is in its earliest stage. When such symptoms are complained of, the patient should be carefully examined, if possible with the sigmoidoscope, as by this means the growth can often be detected at quite an early stage, when removal will be successful.

In the later stages the symptoms are more definite. Pain is more or less constant. It may take the form of occasional sharp attacks of colic, or be of a dull, constant character. When the growth is in the cæcal region, the time at which the pain comes on sometimes bears a relationship to meals, being worse some three or four hours after food. When in the pelvic colon it may have a relationship to defæcation.

The pain is as a rule not well localized, but occasionally may be. Sometimes the patient is conscious of an obstruction at some part of the colon, and will state that he feels there is difficulty in the passage of the bowel contents past a certain point.

Constipation occurs almost always, sooner or later. At first this is easily relieved by aperients; but later, aperients bring on pain, or cause diarrhœa. As a rule, irregularity of the bowels is the condition which first occurs, and later obstruction. Sometimes complete obstruction is the first symptom noticed. In some others it is an attack of partial obstruction due to fæcal impaction. This is relieved satisfactorily by aperients or enemata, and often the true cause of the condition is missed. All cases of fæcal impaction should be carefully examined, as the condition usually results from slight stricturing of the bowel.

As already mentioned, diarrhœa is often an early symptom, and may also occur in the later stages. It is, however, spurious, and careful enquiry will elicit the fact that but little is passed.

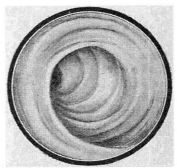

Fig. 63.—Sudden narrowing of the bowel just below a growth in the sigmoid flexure. (The growth was adherent in the left iliac fossa.) (Sigmoidoscopic.)

It is due to the irritation set up by the growth and by the fæces retained above it. Occasionally diarrhœa is a very marked feature of the condition.

Blood in the stools is seldom present in the early stages, and in many cases is absent throughout. Although it is the exception to see blood in the stools, a careful microscopical examination will usually reveal the presence of a few blood corpuscles.

There are two symptoms which are often mentioned as of importance, namely, loss of weight or cachexia, and ribbon or pipe-stem fæces. Neither of these is, however, of any importance or diagnostic value. Loss of weight only occurs in the late stages when there is a large growth, or when diarrhœa is a prominent symptom; and it is commoner in other conditions

OF THE COLON

than in cancer. Pipe-stem fæces can only occur in rectal cancer when the growth involves the anus, as it is obvious that the fæces will take their shape from the *last* orifice through which they pass, and that even if the fæces became narrowed in passing a stricture in the colon, they would be re-moulded in the rectum.

In a few instances the first thing to draw attention to the growth is the presence of a tumour in the abdomen. This is more often the case when the growth is in the cæcal region, as here

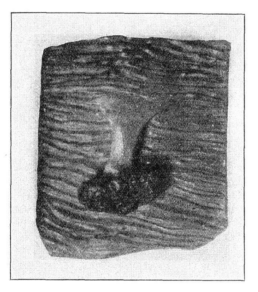

Fig. 64.—An adeno-carcinomatous polypus of the pelvic colon. From a specimen of the author's. The polypus was detected by the sigmoidoscope, and later resected, together with two inches of the colon; the ends being anastomosed. (*Natural size.*)

a growth may reach a considerable size before any symptoms sufficient to draw the patient's attention to his condition have arisen. Although it is fairly easy to make a diagnosis of cancer of the colon when a palpable tumour is present, it is of the utmost importance that the diagnosis should, if possible, be made before this, as by the time a tumour has reached a sufficient size to be palpable the best time for its removal has probably passed.

It cannot be too strongly emphasized that if cancer of the

colon is to be successfully treated, it is necessary that patients should be carefully examined directly there are any symptoms the least suspicious of that condition.

Secondary Results of Cancer of the Colon.—Intestinal obstruction is by far the commonest of these, and may be said to occur in almost all cases. It is often the symptoms of obstruction which first call attention to the disease. The obstruction is never complete, and there is always a slight lumen which will allow fluid contents to pass. In many cases it remains partial for a long period, giving rise to the typical symptoms of chronic obstruction, and resulting in hypertrophy and dilatation of the bowel above the stricture. Sooner or later, however, the narrow opening becomes blocked, either from a hard mass of fæces or a foreign body becoming impacted in it, and acute obstruction then sets in. This may also result from a kink occurring as the result of the growth having become adherent to some other organ or structure, or owing to the mesentery becoming shortened from contraction of the fibrous tissue about the growth. Acute obstruction may also occur from intussusception started by a growth in the colon. The late Mr. Barnard found five cases of this condition in the records of the London Hospital.

Ulceration of the growth does not occur at so early a stage of the disease as in the case of rectal cancer, probably owing to the fact that the colon is not so subjected to injury from the passage of hard fæcal masses.

Spontaneous anastomosis occurred in three of the cases in my series. In two, the transverse colon communicated with the stomach, and in the other with the ileum. Tuttle operated upon two cases, in one of which the sigmoid communicated with the ileum near its termination ; and in the other the two extremities of the sigmoid flexure communicated with each other and shortcircuited the central portion.

As a rule the anastomosis is only a small opening, but sometimes it is large enough to allow most of the intestinal contents to be short-circuited.

The two parts of bowel first become adherent at the base of the growth ; and then the growth extends into the walls of the adherent viscus. Later, ulceration occurs, and the bloodsupply being poorest in the central portion a communication is established between the two. In a few cases, however, the communication occurs differently. The growth in the colon becomes ulcerated, the ulcer perforates the bowel-wall, and a pericolic abscess forms, communicating by the ulcer with the colon. This abscess then becomes adherent to some other viscus, such as the stomach or ileum, and eventually bursts into it and establishes a communication between it and the colon by way of the abscess.

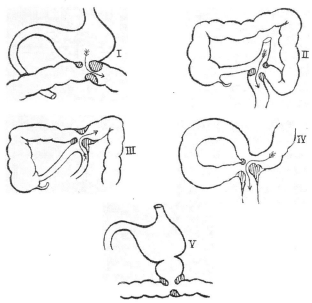

Fig. 65.—Diagrams illustrating different ways in which spontaneous anastomosis may result from a malignant growth in the colon. I.—Anastomosis between stomach and transverse colon. II.—Anastomosis between ileum and sigmoid flexure. III.—Anastomosis between ileum and transverse colon. IV.—Anastomosis between two loops of sigmoid flexure. V.—Anastomosis by abscess formation between stomach and transverse colon.

Malignant peritonitis is very rare as a complication of cancer of the colon.

Acute dilatation of the colon may occur above a malignant stricture. The dilatation may involve the colon immediately above the stricture, or may affect the cæcum only. Thus, the stricture may be in the sigmoid flexure, and the colon between this and the cæcum may be almost normal, and yet extreme dilatation of the cæcum may be found. This is generally a terminal and fatal complication.

Fatal Termination in Cancer of the Colon.—Cancer of the colon seldom kills directly, or even so directly as cancer of most other organs. The fatal termination may occur from one of several secondary consequences. It may be from acute intestinal obstruction; from a toxæmia due to the absorption of poisons in the foul bowel contents retained above the stricture; from acute peritonitis consequent upon a perforating ulcer in the dilated bowel above the growth; or from extensive suppuration due to perforation of the growth or of an ulcer in the bowel above it.

Sarcoma of the Colon.—This is a very rare form of disease of the colon, and I have only been able to find seven cases of the condition. As one would expect, the patients are younger as a rule than is the case with cancer.

The ages in these seven cases were as follows:—

1. Male, age 17.
2. Female ,, 50
3. Male ,, 12
4. Female ,, 21
5. Male, age 8
6. Female ,, not stated
7. ,, ,, 5.

In all these seven cases the growth was in the cæcal region. It is generally a fusiform-celled sarcoma, but in one case it was myxo-sarcoma, and in one a fibro-sarcoma. Sarcoma differs markedly from cancer in appearance, as it looks as if it had invaded the bowel-wall from outside. The mucous membrane is at first intact, and is stretched over the tumour. It originates in the interstitial tissues of the bowel-wall, and tends to spread along the submucous and subperitoneal layers, both circularly and longtitudinally. In cut sections these two layers are seen to be greatly thickened and to consist entirely of sarcomatous tissue. The growth does not affect the mucous membrane early, and it does not tend to ulcerate into the bowel lumen. There was no ulceration in any of these seven cases. In some, the growth seems to spread along the bowel, forming a tubular stricture, and forms outgrowths or tumours under the peritoneum; while in others it tends rather to spread into the bowel and form a large tumour filling up the lumen.

The growth may apparently start in the subperitoneal layer, and in one patient almost the whole growth was outside the muscular coat. It appears to originate in the neighbourhood of the ileocæcal valve, but there is nothing to show exactly where it started. Marked ascites due to involvement of the peritoneum was present in one of the cases.

TREATMENT OF CANCER OF THE COLON.

Cancer of the colon can be very successfully treated by operation, and excellent results can be obtained as regards both the subsequent comfort of the patient and freedom from future recurrence of the tumour.

As has already been pointed out, growths of the colon tend to remain localized to the bowel-wall for a long time, and do not readily give rise to secondary gland-involvement in the root of the mesentery or posterior peritoneal chain of glands. They grow slowly, and but seldom, and only in their later stages, give rise to metastatic deposits in other parts of the body. They do not readily become adherent to important organs, though an exception to this statement must be made in the case of growths of the transverse colon, which frequently involve the stomach. Large portions of the colon can be removed without causing the patient any serious subsequent inconvenience, or preventing him from enjoying life.

The operation for excision of a cancer of the colon does not as a rule present any very serious difficulties, and there are many different methods of dealing with the bowel, after the growth has been excised, which can be adopted according to the exigencies of the case.

The most important factor, as in cancer anywhere else in the body, is early diagnosis. Our methods of diagnosing cancer of the bowel have much improved in recent years, and it is now the exception for a growth to reach a large size before it is recognized. Perhaps fortunately, cancer of the colon draws attention to itself at an early stage by producing obstruction.

In many cases cancer is first detected at an operation undertaken for the relief of obstruction. It will therefore be necessary to consider first the methods of dealing with cases of obstruction of the colon due to cancer, and then to consider the treatment of the growth itself. The actual details of the different operations are considered separately, and I shall deal here only with the indications for operation and the choice of methods.

THE TREATMENT OF OBSTRUCTION DUE TO CANCER OF THE COLON.—Most cases of cancer of the large bowel present themselves to the surgeon with symptoms of obstruction either acute or chronic. When there is acute obstruction, the obvious indications are to relieve the obstruction, which immediately threatens a fatal issue, rather than to excise the growth, which may be dealt with afterwards, and at any rate can only be directly fatal at some later date. The surgeon should not be tempted into doing a complete operation, which, though it may be ideal in theory, is in practice too often attended by fatal consequences.

Patients with acute obstruction of the colon are generally in a profound toxæmic condition owing to the accumulation of poisonous substances in the large bowel, and are not in a state to stand any but the simplest and briefest of operations. Moreover, to excise the growth and anastomose the ends in a patient with acute obstruction, is to leave the patient with a newly-formed joint in the bowel which will certainly be subjected almost immediately to the pressure of the accumulated contents of the bowel above the previous stricture, and this is putting more strain upon the surgeon's handiwork than is at all justifiable. When there is chronic obstruction, but the symptoms are not acute, the choice of method must depend upon whether it is possible entirely to empty the bowel above the stricture. If it is possible by means of aperients to satisfactorily empty the bowel, and the surgeon is certain that there is no accumulation of fæcal material above the growth, then resection of the growth and immediate end-to-end or lateral anastomosis of the bowel would seem justifiable.

But if the bowel cannot be so emptied, the case should be treated in the same way as if acute obstruction existed. This, though it entails the patient undergoing at least two operations, is infinitely safer than performing an anastomosis with accumulated fæces above the line of suture.

I have collected a large number of cases with the view of ascertaining the safest methods of dealing with cases of cancer of the colon, and for this purpose have taken only those in which the growth has been removed either at the first or at some subsequent operation, and have divided these into groups according to the method adopted in each case.

CASES OF IMMEDIATE EXCISION OF THE GROWTH, WITH ANASTOMOSIS OF THE BOWEL, EITHER END-TO-END OR LATERALLY, BY SUTURE.

Cases.	Died.	Recovered.	Percentage Mortality.
86	32	54	37

Six cases recovered with a fæcal fistula.

CASES OF IMMEDIATE EXCISION WITH ANASTOMOSIS BY MURPHY'S BUTTON.

Cases.	Died.	Recovered.	Percentage Mortality.
18	7	11	38

IMMEDIATE EXCISION OF THE GROWTH, THE ENDS OF THE BOWEL BEING BROUGHT OUT OF THE ABDOMEN AND AN ARTIFICIAL ANUS ESTABLISHED. FOLLOWED LATER BY END-TO-END ANASTOMOSIS OR DESTRUCTION OF THE SPUR (PAUL'S METHOD).

Cases.	Died.	Recovered.	Percentage Mortality.
23	4	19	17

CASES IN WHICH AN ARTIFICIAL ANUS WAS MADE AND EXCISION OF THE GROWTH PERFORMED LATER.

Cases.	Died.	Recovered.	Percentage Mortality.
5	0	5	nil.

Moynihan's figures in his book on operations on the abdomen give similar results; they are:—

Immediate excision and anastomosis—3 cases with 1 death.

Paul's operation—12 cases with 1 death.

Colotomy followed by excision—17 cases with 3 deaths.

The above figures show that, while excision with immediate anastomosis is the most popular method, it is attended with by far the highest mortality.

The figures indicate that colotomy followed by excision is safer than excision and bringing the ends out; but several of the cases in my tables were not done by Paul's operation with glass tubes. It seems probable, therefore, that both methods are about equally satisfactory as regards a low mortality.

Immediate excision and anastomosis is attended by more than double the mortality of the operations in which an artificial anus is established; and in spite of its obvious advantages it should certainly not be performed except where the bowel can be completely emptied. The fact that a fæcal fistula occurred in several of the cases that did recover, shows that the line of suture did not hold, and that the patient had run a very serious risk of losing his life.

Paul's operation, in which the growth is excised at the first operation, and the two ends of the bowel are brought out and glass tubes tied into them to form an artificial anus, has the obvious advantage over colotomy followed by excision, that the growth is removed at the earliest possible time. It does not, however, save the patient from a subsequent operation, as a secondary operation to close the artificial anus will almost certainly be necessary. In the case of colotomy followed by excision of the growth, three operations may be necessary, the third being done to close the artificial anus after the growth has been excised and the continuity of the bowel restored. The third operation may be avoided by closing the artificial anus at the second operation; this, however, considerably increases the risk of the second operation. One objection to Paul's method is, that if the growth is to be excised properly, together with its lymphatic area, the operation will in many cases take some time to perform. This sometimes renders it unsuitable where acute obstruction exists at the time. Also, it is, of course, only possible where, after excision of the growth, the two ends of the bowel can easily be brought up to the surface.

An operation for cancer of the colon should aim at excising, not only the growth, but also the whole of the lymphatic area in the mesentery, and, if possible, the chain of glands in the root of the mesentery and along the vessels passing to the affected portion of bowel. This is not a very difficult matter in most parts of the colon, but it often necessitates the sacrifice of a considerable length of gut in order to make certain that the blood-supply to that left behind is good. A large wedge-shaped piece of mesocolon should be removed, and the peritoneum at the back of the abdomen stripped up sufficiently to allow the fat and glands to be cleared out.

As I have already shown in discussing the pathology, growths of the colon spread round the bowel-wall and up and down in the submucous layers, and cancer cells frequently appear in this layer at some little distance from the apparent edge of the growth. Operations, therefore, in which the growth is excised but the bowel is not resected, or in which the bowel is cut close to the growth, are more than likely to fail in eradicating the disease. The entire circumference of the bowel should always be removed, and the gut be divided at least an inch, and if possible more, from the extreme limits of the growth both above and below.

Another plan for dealing with growths in the colon must be mentioned, namely by immediate short-circuit of the growth by lateral anastomosis, followed later by excision and closure of the ends. This method is certainly inferior to those previously mentioned.

Indications for Removing the Growth.—It is too often supposed that because, on opening the abdomen, the growth is found to be large or to be accompanied by a number of enlarged glands, it is therefore useless to remove it. In discussing the pathology it was pointed out that cancer of the colon tends to remain localized for long periods, and that the enlarged glands are frequently not cancerous; they do not, therefore, necessarily mean that the tumour has passed beyond the stage of successful removal, or that if the glands cannot all be removed, rapid recurrence will necessarily follow. Even adhesions are often not cancerous, and if the tumour can be removed and the continuity of the bowel ultimately restored without very serious risk, the operation should most certainly be proceeded with.

There are several instances in which there were enlarged glands in the mesocolon at the time of operation, and yet the patient did not develop any signs of recurrence of the growth. Mr. Charters Symonds records a case in which enlarged glands were left in the mesocolon, but the patient remained free from recurrence ten years later.

Paul records two cases. One, in which glands as large as filberts were present in the root of the mesentery, was well and free from recurrence five years after excision of the growth. In the other case there were also many enlarged glands, but the patient was free from recurrence two-and-a-half years after the operation.

Adhesions of the growth to other viscera should also not necessarily be considered as contraindicating excision, unless the adhesions are to some part which cannot be removed. If they are to the stomach, a portion of the latter viscus can be excised with the tumour. I know two cases in which this was successfully done. Similarly, if the ileum is involved, a portion of it can be resected. In the case of adhesions to the abdominal wall, there is no great difficulty in removing the affected portion, providing it is not too extensive.

Excision of Growths in the Cæcal Region.—These lend themselves readily to extensive resection, as the entire cæcal angle of the colon can be freed and removed together with the growth. Any attempts to resect portions of the cæcum will probably end in failure, both as regards removal of the disease, and also satisfactory restoration of the parts. The peritoneum attaching the cæcum and ascending colon to the posterior abdominal wall should be divided on each side, and the entire cæcal angle stripped up, together with the growth and tissues in the iliac fossa. Next, the vessels should be defined, care being taken to avoid the duodenum, ureter, and spermatic vessels. Those vessels that will require ligature are the ileocolic and cæcal arteries. If there are any glands along the line of the right ileocolic artery, it may be further necessary to ligature the right colic artery which lies close to it, in order to make certain of clearing them away. The entire cæcal angle and tumour can now be easily brought out of the wound. Clamps are next applied to the ileum and colon, and the tumour and cæcum are cut away. If it has been necessary to ligature the right colic artery, the greater part of the ascending colon must also be removed, as its blood-supply has been damaged.

The next step is to deal with the bowel ends. It is most important to see that there is a good blood-supply to the stump of bowel left after division. If this is not satisfactory, more bowel should be resected until an efficient blood-supply is obtained.

The choice of a method must, of course, depend very largely upon the circumstances of the case. It will not always be possible to bring the stump of the ascending colon sufficiently out of the wound to establish an artificial anus by Paul's method. If, however, it is possible to bring up the stump, then a large glass Paul's tube should be tied into it, and a similar tube into the stump of the ileum. These two portions of bowel should then be stitched together over an area of about two inches, to facilitate the use of an enterotome afterwards.

Should it be decided to anastomose the bowel at once, there are two methods available. The stump of the ascending colon can be closed up, and the ileum implanted into its side or into the transverse colon ; or, the stumps may be joined end-to-end by suture, after their respective openings have been made to correspond in size by any of the recognized methods. There is still another method, namely, to close both ends and do a lateral anastomosis, but this has nothing to recommend it, and several disadvantages.

Undoubtedly the best procedure is to close the end of the colon and implant the end of the ileum into it. If much of the ascending colon has been removed it will be necessary to implant the ileum into the transverse colon. Closure of the colon, and lateral implantation of the ileum into it, can be very rapidly done, and makes an excellent joint. Charters Symonds in his Lettsomian Lectures in 1908, advocated using a Murphy's button reinforced with Lembert sutures to make the anastomosis. Stitching, however, is as quick, and certainly a preferable method.

End-to-end anastomosis is more difficult, only applicable in some cases, and much more liable to failure, while it does not seem to have any advantages over lateral implantation.

Owing to the fluid nature of the contents of the ileum, immediate anastomosis is much safer, even when obstruction is present, in cases of cæcal cancer than in cancer of the descending or pelvic colon.

In my collected cases there were sixty-five cases of excision of the cæcum for cancer, with nineteen deaths from the operation.

Cancer of the Hepatic Flexure.—Excision of growths of the hepatic flexure is not often possible, because, there being as a rule no mesentery, the growth early becomes adherent posteriorly. In my series there is only one instance of successful resection of a growth of the hepatic flexure, and in this case there was rapid recurrence.

Cancer of the Transverse Colon.—Excision of growths in this situation is not especially difficult, as this portion of the colon can be drawn out of the abdominal cavity. In my series there are five cases of excision of a growth in the transverse colon. In one, an artificial anus was first established above the growth, and, later on, the growth was excised and the bowel joined by sutures; the patient recovered. In one case Paul's method was adopted; and in the three others the growth was excised, and the colon joined end-to-end by sutures at once. In two of the cases the stomach was involved in the growth, and an elliptical portion of this viscus was excised, together with the growth. Four recovered. The case that died was one in which immediate end-to-end anastomosis was performed. In another of the cases of immediate end-to-end union, a fæcal fistula formed after the operation.

Cancer of the Splenic Flexure—There are two cases in which excision was performed. In one the bowel was anastomosed end-to-end by suture; the patient died. In the other the transverse colon was united to the sigmoid flexure; this patient recovered, but a fæcal fistula formed.

Cancer of the Sigmoid Flexure—In by far the majority of cases of cancer of the colon the growth is in the sigmoid flexure. With the exception of those at the extreme lower end, these growths may be readily excised, owing to the mobility of this part of the colon. The sigmoid flexure is, however, not so suitable for end-to-end anastomosis after excision as the cæcal angle, owing to the fact that the fæcal contents are more solid, and the suture line will be subjected to a greater strain after operation. Paul's operation is undoubtedly the safest method of dealing with growths in this situation. The mortality from it in growths of the sigmoid is very low indeed. Paul himself has performed it a great many times, with only one or two deaths.

M. J. Boselius states that out of twenty-eight cases operated upon by this method in the Breslau Hospital there were only four deaths; whereas formerly, when end-to-end union was performed, the mortality was fifty per cent. Hochenegg had only one death in fourteen cases.

In my series there are five resections of the sigmoid for cancer with immediate end-to-end anastomosis; of these, four died from the operation. Eight were treated by Paul's method, or by the establishment of an artificial anus previous to excision, and of these none died. There can be no doubt, therefore, that in spite of the obvious disadvantages of a temporary artificial anus and of a double operation, the best method of dealing with the bowel after excision of a growth in the sigmoid is to bring the ends out and establish an artificial anus, this being subsequently closed by a second operation. This operation does not incur much more danger than a simple colotomy. Colotomy above the growth, followed by excision, has the serious disadvantage that there is considerable danger of not getting the surface of the abdomen clean enough for the second operation, and a risk of soiling the peritoneum during its performance.

In excising a growth of the sigmoid flexure care should be taken to go well wide of the growth (at least an inch on each side of it, and preferably more), and to make a clean sweep of the mesocolon containing the lymphatics, and the portion of bowel in which the tumour is situated. The peritoneum can be stripped up over the iliac vessels if necessary, and any glands in this situation removed. The glands, if present, will probably be found lying close to the sigmoid and inferior mesenteric arteries. Mr. Moynihan states that there is always a gland situated on the inferior mesenteric artery, and that the greater part of the sigmoid loop, the mesocolon, and the inferior mesenteric artery must be removed entirely. This makes the operation a very extensive one, and, although it has been shown that after ligature of the inferior mesenteric artery there is still an adequate blood-supply to the parts that remain, such an extensive operation seems hardly necessary in all cases in view of the fact that other observers have not found this enlarged gland on the vessel to be by any means invariably present. The presence of glands along the inferior mesenteric artery should be looked for, and such

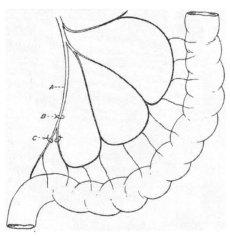

Fig. 66.—A, Inferior mesenteric artery; B, ligature without destroying anastomosis; C, ligatures breaking the anastomosis. [JAMIESON and DOBSON, *Proc. Roy. Soc. Med.*, Vol. 2, 1909.]

extensive removal only carried out if they are discovered, though, even when enlarged, it does not necessarily follow that the gland is carcinomatous.

Considerable difficulty exists when the growth, as is not infrequently the case, is situated just above the recto-sigmoidal junction. When the growth is here it will be so deeply situated in the pelvis that considerable difficulty may be experienced in removing it; but by using the Trendelenburg position, and freely incising the peritoneum at the front and sides of the growth, it can always be removed. The chief trouble is experienced in dealing with the bowel afterwards. There are three alternatives :—

1. To close or pack off the upper end of the rectum, and to bring the stump of the sigmoid out of the abdomen and form an artificial anus.

2. To remove the entire rectum and bring the stump of the sigmoid down to the anus.

3. To anastomose the ends by means of a tube tied into the sigmoid and passed down through the rectum and out of the anus.

The first method has the objection that it leaves the patient with a permanent artificial anus; while the second involves a most formidable operation and sacrifices a normal rectum.

The third method gives quite satisfactory results, and enables the continuity of the bowel to be restored in cases where end-to-end anastomosis is impossible. It will be described in detail later.

Summary.

1. In cases where acute obstruction is present at the time of operation, a temporary artificial anus should always be made, and excision of the growth postponed till a later time; or the growth should be excised and the ends of the bowel brought out.

2. Unless the bowel above the growth can be entirely emptied before operation, an artificial anus should be established before proceeding to excise the growth; or Paul's operation be done.

3. In excising the growth, the bowel should always be resected, and *at least* an inch of normal bowel removed on each side of the growth.

4. Whenever possible the lymphatic area should be cleared with the growth; but inability to do this is not necessarily a bar to successful removal.

5. Immediate end-to-end anastomosis after excision may be performed in dealing with the right half of the colon, but is dangerous on the left side.

6. Paul's operation, or colotomy followed by excision, is by far the safest operation when excising growths of the sigmoid.

7. The presence of enlarged glands, or adhesions to other structures, should not necessarily be taken as contra-indicating resection, providing removal is possible.

Recurrence of the Growth after Excision.—Owing to the fact that cancer of the colon tends to remain localized for long periods, and but seldom gives rise to metastatic deposits, recurrence after operation is not very common. I have not collected a series of statistics to show the frequency of recurrence, because owing to the widely different operations performed by surgeons, and in different cases, any such statistics would be valueless. Until a more or less uniform operation becomes recognized in excising growths of the colon, such statistics can hardly be of much value. I have, however, been able to find many records of cases in which the patient, after resection of a growth from the colon, has remained free from recurrence for long periods.

Mr. Symonds has recorded a case in which the patient, after a growth in the ileocæcal angle had been resected, remained free from recurrence ten years later. Mr. Paul records two cases free from recurrence six and five years respectively after excision. Mr. Clogg records two cases six and four years after operation and free from recurrence. Mr. Moynihan records two cases remaining well seven years after operation; and nine cases well three years after. Boselius records four cases free from recurrence five years after operation. These are sufficient to show that very long periods of freedom from recurrence may be obtained after resection of the colon for cancer.

Palliative Operations.—Even when the growth cannot be removed, much may be done by the performance of a suitable operation to render the patient more comfortable and prolong his life. The operations that may be performed for this purpose are:—

1. Excision of as much of the growth as can be got away.
2. Short-circuiting the growth.
3. Making an artificial anus above the growth.

Some surgeons have advised that, even when it is found at the operation that there are glands which cannot be removed, or metastatic deposits in the liver, the best plan is still to excise the primary growth, and that this will give the patient a longer lease of life than short-circuiting. There is a good deal to be said for this view, and always the possibility that the glands which are not removed are not cancerous. If the primary growth can be easily removed without much danger to the patient, this is probably the best treatment; but it does not seem right to subject the patient to a dangerous and prolonged operation if there are secondary deposits already present which

MALIGNANT DISEASE

cannot be removed. Short-circuiting the growth is undoubtedly the best method when it is found that excision is impossible. It does away with the danger of obstruction, and does not leave the patient with the discomforts of a colotomy.

If the growth is in the cæcum, the ileum should be divided, the cæcal end closed, and the proximal end implanted into the ascending or transverse colon. This gives a better result, and is just as easily performed as lateral anastomosis in this

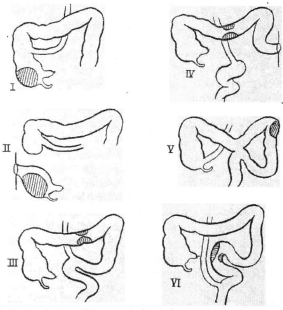

Fig. 67.—Diagram showing different methods of short-circuiting a tumour of the colon. I.—Ileum implanted after division into ascending colon. II.—Ditto, but cæcum excluded and opening by fistula on skin surface. III.—Ileo-sigmoidostomy after dividing ileum. IV.—Ditto, and exclusion of colon with fistula to skin. V.—Transverse colon anastomosed to sigmoid. VI.—Ileo-sigmoidostomy for growth in colon.

situation. Ileo-colostomy by lateral implantation seems to be the best operation for growths in the right half of the colon, and in the transverse colon. An even better operation, probably, is to divide the colon above the anastomosis and bring the excluded portion to the skin, as this does away with the possibility of fæces accumulating in the excluded portion of the colon; it has, however, the disadvantage of leaving the patient with a fistulous opening. When the growth is in the left side of the colon, the choice lies between lateral anastomosis between the transverse colon and sigmoid and ileo-sigmoidostomy. In a few cases where the growth is in the centre of the sigmoid loop, lateral anastomosis between the two limbs of the loop will be suitable.

Colotomy is the only available method when the growth is situated too low down in the sigmoid to allow of the ileum being anastomosed below it. It is also not safe to perform short-circuiting if obstruction is present at the time of operation, and this must often be the case. Colotomy must then be done ; or, preferably, a fæcal fistula established above the growth, and a short-circuiting operation performed after the obstruction has been relieved, the fæcal fistula being then allowed to close.

In conclusion, it must be borne in mind, when a tumour of the colon is discovered, that it may be a case of hyperplastic tuberculosis, and not cancer. Short of cutting open the tumour it is impossible to make a certain diagnosis between these two conditions, and in view of this possibility the tumour should either be excised or short-circuited if it can be managed ; for if the case is one of tubercle, recovery will very probably follow either of these operations ; whereas, if the surgeon closes the abdomen under the impression that he is dealing with a hopeless case of cancer, the patient will almost certainly die.

Chapter XIX.

TRAUMATISM.

The colon is so deeply situated in the abdominal cavity, and so well protected, that, apart from gross injury involving the whole or greater part of the abdominal viscera, it is but rarely the seat of severe traumatism.

Rupture of the colon from direct violence is a very rare condition, and but few instances have been recorded. Out of 292 cases of abdominal injuries collected by Mr. Makins at St. Thomas' Hospital in nine years, the intestine was injured in 22, and in only 5 of these was the colon involved.

It requires a very serious traumatism to rupture the colon, and in most of the cases the cause is either a crush such as will result from being run over by a heavy vehicle, or a severe blow such as the kick in the abdomen by a horse.

One would suppose that the transverse colon, where it passes across the spinal column, would be the part most likely to be thus ruptured. The cases I have been able to collect are too few to warrant any conclusions on this point, but at least it may be stated that the transverse colon is not alone affected, for in two instances the ascending colon was ruptured as the result of direct traumatism of the abdomen.

The nature of the injury of the colon varies considerably, from a complete tear or tears involving the whole lumen of the bowel, to a minute opening. In some, the colon was apparently not ruptured at the time of the accident, but was so damaged that it gave way in one or more places later.

In a case recorded by Mr. Battle, the rupture occurred at the splenic flexure as the result of the patient being run over, and the tear was apparently mainly post-peritoneal.

Rupture of the colon from within must be an extremely rare

condition, but I have been able to find two instances. In both the nature of the accident was similar. In one, the patient, a man, fell off a step-ladder on to an umbrella stand, and the handle of an umbrella entered the rectum and was broken off. It found its way into the transverse colon and perforated the bowel-wall. The umbrella handle, which measured 7 inches in length, was subsequently removed by operation from the transverse colon, and the patient made a good recovery. In the other case, the patient fell upon a broom handle, which passed up the rectum and perforated the bowel just above the recto-sigmoidal junction. The patient was operated on a few hours later, when a large rent was found in the anterior wall of the bowel. It was closed with stitches, and the patient recovered.

Rupture of the colon from indirect violence must be extremely rare, but McCaskey has recorded a case in which the splenic flexure ruptured as the result of violent peristalsis above a stricture of the sigmoid flexure.

As a rule, in a rupture of the colon the injury is complicated by severe bruising or laceration of the neighbouring bowel, or of the mesentery. Surgical emphysema, owing to the escape of intestinal gas from the bowel into the subperitoneal areolar tissue, has been present in some of the cases.

TREATMENT.

If the severity and nature of the injury can be diagnosed, there should be no hesitation in resorting to immediate operation. The indications for operating are the same as for perforation of the bowel in any part.

It will be but seldom that the exact nature and site of the lesion can be diagnosed. As a rule, all that can be known is that a serious injury to some portion of the bowel has occurred. Under these circumstances a median incision will be indicated, so as to allow the whole of the bowel to be examined. When the rent has been discovered, it will depend upon the nature of the lesion as to what procedure is adopted. If there is only a small rent, and the neighbouring bowel-wall is not seriously damaged, simple closure of the tear by Lembert sutures is all that is necessary, combined with careful cleansing of the peritoneal cavity, drainage being provided for if any serious soiling has occurred. If the colon is completely torn across, or if the bowel-wall has been so damaged as to negative any hope of its recovery, resection of the damaged portion will have to be performed. The bowel may either be united end-to-end by suture, or the ends can be closed and the bowel united by lateral anastomosis. In the case of the transverse colon or sigmoid flexure, the ends of the colon can be brought out of the abdomen after resection and sutured to the skin so as to form an artificial anus; the spur may be destroyed later on and the opening closed by plastic operation, or an anastomosis performed at some later period when the patient has recovered from the shock of the injury.

The exact character of the operative procedure must, however, vary in different cases according to the nature of the injury and the condition of the patient.

Considering the serious nature of the injury in these cases, and the difficulty of making a correct diagnosis before peritonitis has developed, the results of operation appear most encouraging. Thus, out of six cases of rupture of the colon submitted to operation, four recovered and two died, while of the cases not operated upon both died.

The following curious case of rupture of the mesosigmoid from direct violence seems worth recording :—

Case.—The patient was a man, aged 20, under the care of Dr. Ross in the German Hospital, New York. He was struck in the abdomen during a fight. Shortly afterwards severe pain in the abdomen induced him to come into the hospital. On admission a mass could be felt in the right iliac fossa, and he was much collapsed. The abdominal muscles were rigid. Immediate operation was decided upon. An intravenous injection was given prior to operation, as the patient was in bad condition. On opening the peritoneum much free blood escaped. There was no rupture of the intestine, but an extensive hæmorrhage between the layers of the mesentery, and the outer layer of the mesosigmoid was denuded of its serous coat for about 4 inches. There was also much blood behind the peritoneum. The serous coat of the mesosigmoid was sutured with fine silk. Two pieces of gauze were packed in to stop the oozing from the mesenteric wound. A fæcal fistula formed on the eighth day from the pressure of the gauze upon a portion of badly nourished bowel. The fistula healed spontaneously on the sixteenth day. The patient left the hospital well on the forty-fifth day, but returned six days later with pain in the abdomen and vomiting. He also stated that his bowels had not been open for twenty-four hours. He was supposed to be suffering from chronic obstruction, and it was thought advisable to operate. At the second operation the old scar was excised. The sigmoid and small bowel were found to be matted together in numerous places. The adhesions were broken up, but in doing so the serous coat was damaged in several places, and in one place an opening was made in the bowel which had to be sewn up. The patient died on the third day after the second operation. The cause of death was general peritonitis.

Chapter XX

COLOTOMY.

The object of this operation is to make an artificial outlet for the fæces, either temporarily or permanently, by establishing an opening between the skin surface and some portion of the colon.

In the pre-Listerian days, when surgeons were afraid to open the peritoneal cavity, lumbar colotomy was always performed when it was necessary to make an artificial anus; but since the introduction of antiseptic methods it has fallen into disuse, and has now with a few exceptions been entirely replaced by inguinal trans-peritoneal colotomy.

This is an operation which at the present day is practically unattended by any mortality. The following is the only instance I have met with in which a fatal result was caused by the operation :—

Case.—I was called one day to see an elderly man who had symptoms of intestinal obstruction. He was suffering from inoperable cancer of the rectum, and five days previously a left inguinal colotomy had been performed by another surgeon. The colotomy had been done by the stitch method, and appeared quite satisfactory; but although the bowel had been opened and aperients given, there had been no action of the bowels, and symptoms of acute obstruction had developed. A cæcostomy was done, but the patient died before the operation could be completed. Post mortem it was discovered, on opening the abdomen in the middle line, that a portion of the great omentum had been caught up in the colotomy stitch in such a way that it dragged upon the centre of the transverse colon, and had formed a sharp kink which entirely obstructed the bowel.

We must, of course, not confuse the mortality due to diseased conditions for which the operation is performed with that due to the operation itself. In many cases it is performed in an attempt to save the life of a patient who is *in extremis,* and in such cases it not infrequently happens that the patient dies in

COLOTOMY

spite of the operation. Colotomy should in skilled hands be almost free from risk.

The usual method of performing colotomy at the present day is to make a small vertical incision through the abdominal wall about half way between the umbilicus and the left anterior superior spine of the ilium. Through this opening a loop of sigmoid is pulled out. The bowel is then pulled down until that portion nearest to the descending colon which can be made to reach the opening is found, and this portion is used to form

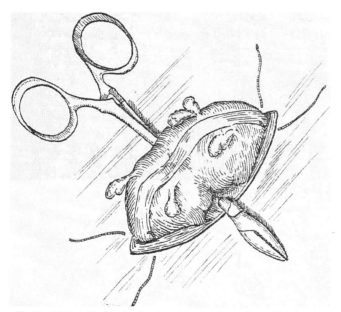

Fig. 68.—Method of performing inguinal colotomy, using a clip to form the spur.

the colotomy. A spur is now made, either by means of a mattress stitch passed through the mesosigmoid, or preferably by a glass rod or a clip which is passed through the mesosigmoid and allowed to rest on the skin on each side of the wound. A stitch is passed through the skin at the end of the incision, and through the anterior longitudinal muscle band. Such a stitch should be inserted at both ends of the wound, to anchor the bowel and prevent any further prolapse. Unless a large incision has been made, one stitch at each end should be sufficient. If there are any large appendices epiploicæ they should be ligatured and removed.

In many text-books the position for the incision is given as the junction of the middle and outer thirds of a line between the umbilicus and the left anterior superior spine. While this incision is directly over the colon, it has the disadvantage that afterwards, when a cup has to be fitted over the colotomy opening, the edge of the cup tends to ride up on the iliac crest as the patient walks or moves, and this results in leakage and discomfort.

I prefer to make the incision much nearer the middle of the abdomen, and far enough away from the pubes and iliac crest to

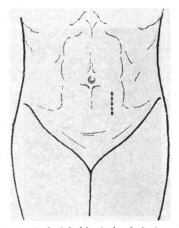

Fig. 69.—Author's incision for inguinal colotomy.

insure that any apparatus afterwards fitted will rest entirely on the abdominal wall. The incision is made through the outer fibres of the rectus muscle, and the bowel pulled out between the muscle fibres. This assists considerably in giving subsequent control.

It is important to make the abdominal wound small, as the resulting control is better. An incision one-and-a-half inches long is sufficient. The bowel is usually opened on the second day after operation. For this purpose no anæsthetic is required, the bowel being quite insensitive. A small transverse cut should be made with a pair of scissors in such a way as to partly divide the bowel. A transverse incision is better than a longitudinal one, because the bleeding is less.

If it is necessary to open the bowel at once, a Paul's tube should be tied into it to prevent soiling of the wound. Some six or eight days later the bowel is completely divided by cutting it across. The whole bowel should be completely divided by inserting one blade of the scissors along the track of the glass rod or clip, and the other outside the bowel, cutting through all the intervening tissue. At the same time, any bowel projecting above the skin level should be trimmed off close to the skin. No anæsthetic is necessary. One of the chief difficulties in securing control over the opening after such an operation is the lack of any sensation which can warn the patient that the bowel is acting. As I have shown in discussing the physiology of the colon, a certain amount of sensation at the opening usually develops in course of time. In such cases the sensory nerves doubtless grow into the mucous membrane from the skin, and it is therefore important to see that there is not a redundant fold of mucosa outside the skin, as the mucous membrane never becomes sensitive for more than a short distance from the skin edge (see diagrams, page 16).

Several new methods of performing colotomy have been devised with the object of giving the patient better control over the opening. The earliest of these consisted in giving a twist to the bowel above the opening, or in stricturing it by means of a ligature; these, however, did not prove satisfactory, and have been abandoned. Witzel was the first to suggest making a valvular opening in the abdominal wall. This was done as follows: A loop of sigmoid colon was first brought out through the usual colotomy incision, and another smaller incision was made below the pelvic brim. A space was then opened up between these two incisions by separating the internal and external oblique muscles, and the loop of bowel was dragged through this space and stitched to the skin at the lower opening, the upper opening being completely closed.

Bailey's modification of this method consists in opening up a space between the skin and external oblique muscle, and bringing the colon out through an incision just above Poupart's ligament.

Tuttle describes a modification of these methods as follows: The ordinary incision is made, and a loop of colon pulled out. This should come outside for at least two inches. The lower fibres of the external oblique are then pulled downward, and the internal oblique is split laterally to the extent of about ¾ of an inch. A canal is next made between the skin and external oblique, downward for 2 inches, and made to open through the skin just above Poupart's ligament. This canal should be large enough to admit the loop of colon easily. By means of a tape and dressing-forceps the end of the loop of bowel is drawn through the lateral slit in the external oblique, and downward through the canal outside this muscle until it emerges at the skin opening. It is held here by stitches or a glass rod, and the abdominal wound is closed in layers (see *Fig.* 70).

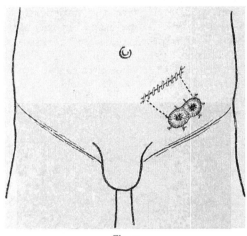

Fig. 70.

It is claimed for these methods that, by wearing a truss which presses upon the skin over the bowel where it passes subcutaneously, the patient obtains complete control over both gas and fæces. The opening, however, is placed in a very inconvenient position in the fold of the groin, and the author's experience of these methods has been that the control is little if any better than that obtained by bringing the bowel straight through the abdominal wall. The valvular opening is good at first, but in a very short time the tension of the bowel straightens out the canal, and if one puts one's finger into the opening it is found to pass straight through the abdominal wall, and all

COLOTOMY

resemblance to a valve has disappeared. The author believes that the best control is obtained by making a small incision and bringing the bowel out through the split fibres of the rectus muscle. When the patient is standing or walking the rectus will be contracted, and will effectually close the opening and prevent leakage. Moreover, at any time, by contracting his recti, he can to a considerable extent prevent leakage from the opening. I have found that patients with this form of colotomy quickly obtain most excellent control, and are able, with little or no trouble, to keep themselves clean.

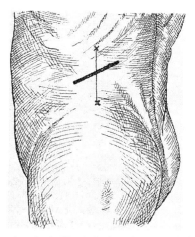

Fig. 71.—Diagram to show the incision for lumbar colotomy. The incision is made with its centre on a line drawn from the tip of the last rib to a point half-an-inch behind the centre of the crest of the ileum.

Lumbar Colotomy.—This, formerly the favourite operation, is now only employed in special cases : as, for instance, when the colon cannot for some reason be brought up to the abdominal wall, and inguinal colotomy is therefore impossible. Right lumbar colotomy is also sometimes performed in place of cæcostomy, as the control afterwards is better owing to the more solid nature of the fæces in the ascending colon.

The patient is laid upon his side, with a firm cushion or sandbag under the loin, in order to flex the trunk sideways and open out the space between the last rib and the iliac crest. The position of the colon is indicated by a vertical line drawn upwards from a point half-an-inch behind the mid-point between the anterior and posterior superior spines of the ilium.

An oblique incision is made, with its centre over this line, and midway between the last rib and the crest of the ilium. The incision should be about 3 inches long. The anterior edge of the quadratus lumborum should be exposed in the back of the incision and, if necessary, partly divided. The wound is then opened until the transversalis fascia is met with. On dividing this, the cellular tissue and fat are seen, and when these are separated, the back of the colon will be exposed in the bottom of the wound. The colon is pulled up into the wound and fixed to the skin by sutures all round, an oval surface of colon being left exposed. If it should be necessary to open the colon at once, a Paul's tube or one of the author's rubber tubes should be tied in, otherwise the colon is opened by a longitudinal incision at the end of twenty-four hours.

If the colon is found to have a mesentery, and it is not possible to expose it extraperitoneally, the peritoneum should be opened in front of the colon and the bowel brought out in the same way as in performing inguinal colotomy. The colon is more likely to have a mesentery on the right than on the left side.

Control over the Opening after Colotomy.—Very pessimistic opinions are generally expressed as regards the comfort of patients upon whom colotomy has been performed. With the object of ascertaining whether such a view is justified I investigated the after-histories of several of the patients upon whom I had performed inguinal colotomy; I found that in old people, especially of the poorer classes, who have but few facilities for keeping themselves clean, there is usually no control over the discharge from the opening. This is more particularly the case with men, and with patients suffering from an exhausting illness, such as cancer of the rectum.

Where, however, the patient was of a better class, and was willing and able to take a little trouble, very good control over the opening was usually obtained; so that I found many patients able to live an ordinary life, mixing with other people and attending to their business without difficulty and without others knowing of their disability.

Some patients had quite a surprising amount of control. One was a man of 33, with a left inguinal colotomy which had been made over a year previously. After the first four months he was always able to tell when the bowels were about to act, and the opening did not cause him the slightest trouble except on one occasion after he had eaten something which disagreed with him. He attended to his business and played football for his local team.

Another patient was a gentleman who lived in the country and hunted several times a week; the colotomy had been done some years previously.

One patient, a stevedore at the London Docks, who had a permanent colotomy, was 62 years of age, and returned to his employment after the operation and worked his eight hours a day. He assured me that the colotomy opening did not interfere with his work, and he was quite able to keep himself clean.

The best control was obtained where there was a small opening without prolapse of the mucous membrane, and when the patient wore a celluloid cup over the opening.

The use of a plug fitting into the opening prevents any sensation being acquired which will warn the patient of the necessity of attention.

A case is recorded by Dr. Mitchell of a woman who was successfully delivered of a child ten months after colotomy had been performed.

Colotomy by Paul's Method.—This is frequently the best and safest method of dealing with the bowel after resection of part of the colon.

The colon is exposed and brought out of the wound in the same way as in performing inguinal colotomy. The wound having been first shut off by gauze packing, the colon is divided, and a Paul's glass tube of suitable size tied into either end by a silk ligature. The two portions of colon are then sewn together side by side, for about two inches of their length, with silk sutures, with the object of ensuring the walls being in contact later, when the enterotome is used (See *Fig.* 72).

The tubes come away in about a week, and some three weeks later the spur is destroyed by means of an enterotome (see page 292). After the spur has been destroyed, the continuity of the bowel is re-established, but a fæcal fistula still remains, which in course of time usually closes of itself; but it may be many months before this occurs, and it is better as a rule to close it by operation. If the spur has been well divided, all that is necessary is to dissect the mucous membrane off the skin and sew it up.

COLOTOMY

There is no necessity to open the peritoneal cavity, and the risk of the operation is therefore slight.

This method of dealing with the bowel after resection of the colon for stenosis or tumour has the disadvantage that the patient has the discomforts of a fæcal fistula for some time, and that a second operation is rendered necessary. On the other hand, there can be no question but that it is by far the safest method. It is practically unattended by any mortality, while immediate end-to-end union is followed by a high death-rate.

Cases in which it is impossible to perform Colotomy.— At times this operation has to be abandoned, either because

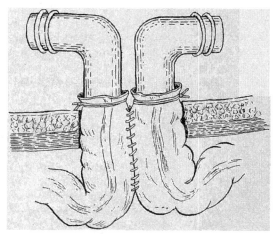

Fig. 72.—Paul's method of performing colotomy.

the colon cannot be found, or because it cannot be made to reach the skin. Such cases are of considerable interest, as they cause great difficulty to the surgeon. They are now less common than in the days when lumbar colotomy was the usual operation. Thus a case is recorded by Lockwood, in which right lumbar colotomy could not be performed because the cæcum and ascending colon lay on the left side of the abdomen. With inguinal colotomy, abnormalities of the colon are less likely to lead to inability to perform the operation, though they may cause considerable difficulty.

The sigmoid flexure being situated on the right side of the

abdomen instead of the left may create difficulty, and this condition is not very uncommon. I have met with one case in which the operation had to be abandoned owing to the sigmoid being fixed in the right iliac fossa. The bowel could not be found on the left side, and on making an incision on the right, it was found to be impossible to bring the sigmoid into the wound.

In two cases the operation was impossible from the fact that the entire colon was fixed and immovable. In both these cases there was hyperplastic tuberculosis of the colon, and cæcostomy had to be done.

Cæcostomy.—This operation is performed when it is not possible to perform colotomy, or when a colotomy opening will not be above the seat of obstruction. It is also sometimes done to deflect the fæcal current from the colon in cases of ulcerative colitis.

The cæcum is exposed through an oblique incision, the centre of which lies over a point half way between the umbilicus and the right anterior superior spine of the ileum. The anterior wall of the cæcum is drawn out of the wound and sewn to the skin and aponeurosis all round the edges of the wound. The stitches should take up the peritoneal and muscular coats only, and when they are all inserted the peritoneal cavity should be completely shut off, and an oval area of the cæcal wall about $1\frac{1}{2}$ in. long should alone remain exposed. Two sutures to act as guides should be inserted into the cæcal wall, and two days later the cæcum is opened by cutting between these guide sutures with a knife. Another method of performing cæcostomy, and a preferable one if the cæcum has to be opened at once, is to enclose a small circular area of the cæcal wall about $\frac{1}{2}$ in. in diameter in a purse-string suture. This portion of the cæcal wall is then held up by an assistant, and a small incision into the cæcum is made in the centre of the circular area; through this one end of a Paul's tube is pushed, and the purse-string suture is then tied firmly on to the tube. The cæcal wall is stitched into the wound and the latter closed, leaving the Paul's tube projecting.

Owing to the liquid nature of the contents of the cæcum, the control over this opening is very unsatisfactory, and the surrounding skin often becomes sore and excoriated. This may to some extent be prevented by keeping the parts well greased with lanolin.

CLOSURE OF A FÆCAL FISTULA OR ARTIFICIAL ANUS BY OPERATION.

A Fæcal Fistula.—The surgeon may be called upon to close a fæcal fistula which has resulted from disease of the colon, or which he or some other surgeon has made, but which is no longer necessary. Operations for closing fæcal fistulæ in the colon are often very difficult, and have not infrequently been attended by a fatal result.

Very careful consideration is advisable before attempting an operation of this nature; it is not justifiable to risk the patient's life for what in many cases is only an inconvenience. Providing the normal channel to the anus is patent and not seriously obstructed, most fæcal fistulæ will close spontaneously if given sufficient time.

The most difficult fistulæ to close are those which communicate with the cæcum. The reasons for this are probably the fluid nature of the contents of the cæcum, and more especially the pressure to which any join in the cæcal wall will be subjected owing to antiperistalsis in the right side of the colon. In some cases several operations have had to be performed before a fæcal fistula in the cæcum could be made to close. The following table, compiled by the author, shows the results of 36 operations undertaken for this purpose or the closure of an artificial anus :—

TABLE OF THE RESULTS OF OPERATIONS FOR THE CLOSURE OF FÆCAL FISTULÆ.

Opening closed successfully	16
First operation failed to close the opening	9
Repeated operations failed	6
Patient died as a result of the operation	5
	36

One of the chief difficulties in operating to close a fæcal fistula is the great danger of the wound becoming infected during the operation. The best plan is to disinfect the fistula, either with cautery or with some powerful antiseptic, and then to dissect out a piece of skin containing the fistula and the entire fistula itself down to the colon; the fistula can then be cut off, and the stump invaginated into the bowel with a purse-string suture (this method is only applicable to very small fistulæ or those leading into the cæcum). Another method is to excise the portion of bowel containing the fistula and carefully close the wound in the bowel with a double row of sutures, the first row taking up all the coats, and the second the peritoneal and muscular coats only. If this is likely to cause serious narrowing of the bowel lumen, the wound in the bowel should be sewn up transversely instead of longitudinally.

Still another plan is to resect that portion of the colon containing the fistula and anastomose the ends. This, however, is attended with much more risk than the previous methods. The success of the operation in any case depends upon very careful asepsis and close stitching.

Where the fistula is associated with stenosis of the colon, there are three methods which have been used for getting rid of it :—

1. The portion of bowel with which the fistula communicates may be resected, together with the stenosis or tumour.

2. It may be short-circuited.

3. It may be excluded, either partially or totally.

If resection is decided upon, it is advisable to perform a preliminary short-circuiting operation ; this can be done without interfering with the fistula, and therefore without danger of infecting the peritoneum.

Short-circuiting will often result in closure of the fæcal fistula. Both partial and total exclusion will almost certainly fail to do this, but they will very materially diminish the discharge therefrom, and greatly increase the patient's comfort.

Artificial Anus.—The closure of a colotomy opening will depend very largely upon the manner in which the original operation was performed. When a temporary colotomy opening has been made by the method described on page 281, with a glass rod or clip, and the bowel has not been completely divided, but only opened on its anterior aspect, it can be quite easily closed without opening the peritoneal cavity. The cut edges of the wound in the colon are first dissected free, and freshened by cutting away the extreme edges. They are then brought back into position, and the wound in the colon is closed by suturing the edges carefully together, a second row of sutures being inserted over the first to make all tight. The colon, being now closed again, is dissected away from its attachments to the abdominal wall until the peritoneum is reached. This is not opened, but is stripped from the underside of the abdominal wall for about an inch all round the opening, or sufficiently far to give the colon a free lumen without kinking. Lastly, the wound in the abdominal wall is closed over the colon (see *Fig.* 73). The portion of colon which originally formed the colotomy is thus left in the subperitoneal tissue, and, if leakage should occur, it will be externally. This method can also be used when the gut has been completely divided. The ends of the colon are freshened, then anastomosed by suture, and lastly buried in the subperitoneal tissue.

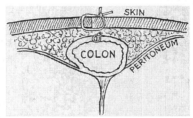

Fig. 73.—Method of closing a colotomy opening extra-peritoneally

It is perhaps unnecessary to point out that, previous to any such operation, the colon should be well cleared by aperients, and steps taken afterwards to prevent any but quite liquid fæces passing through it for the next ten days.

Another plan of closing a colotomy opening without exposing the peritoneal cavity is that used after colotomy by Paul's method. This is also applicable to a colotomy opening made in the ordinary manner.

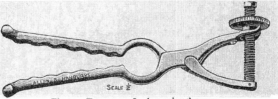

Fig. 74.—Enterotome for destroying the spur.

The spur between the two portions of bowel is first destroyed, so as to make the upper and lower limbs of the colon communicate freely below the skin level. This is done by means of an enterotome ; or a clip forceps with long blades will do equally well.

The surgeon places his first and second fingers into the two openings of the colon, and assures himself that there is nothing but the respective walls of the two portions of colon lying between his fingers. The two blades of the enterotome are then inserted along his fingers so that one blade lies in each portion of bowel, and the instrument is closed so as to grip tightly the spur over a distance of about 1½ to 2 inches. The instrument having been firmly fixed in position, and the handles supported by dressings, it is left until it comes loose owing to the destruction of the spur by sloughing. The blades of the instrument are very apt to slip up the spur, and it may be necessary to re-apply it several times.

If any of the mesentery is included between the blades, and sometimes when it is not, there is a considerable amount of pain while the enterotome is cutting its way through, and for this it will be necessary to give morphia.

It takes as a rule, from two to five days to destroy the spur and join up the two portions of bowel. If the bowel is examined after the enterotome has become loose, it will be found that there is some swelling of the edges of the opening, but this disappears in a few days. The fæces will at once begin to pass in part by the normal channel, and steps can then be taken to close the skin opening. This necessitates an anæsthetic. The edges of the mucous membrane should be dissected loose from the skin and muscles, turned in, and stitched together. The skin, and as much of the deep parts as possible, should then be brought together above, so as to close the skin opening.

If the spur is freely divided with the enterotome, the external opening will close itself in time ; but this may take many months. This is a very safe, though rather tedious, method of closing a colotomy opening.

Chapter XXI.

APPENDICOSTOMY AND VALVULAR CÆCOSTOMY.

APPENDICOSTOMY.

This operation was first performed by Weir, of America, in a case of ulcerative colitis.

It was the outcome of a suggestion by Dr. Hale White in 1895, that a right inguinal colotomy should be done in cases of intractable colitis.

Weir's original operation proved extraordinarily successful. The patient rapidly recovered as the result of daily irrigation of the colon, whereas previously the only satisfactory results in similar cases had been obtained by establishing an artificial anus on the right side, a procedure almost as objectionable as the disease. Weir's first operation was performed in 1902, and since then it has been done in a considerable number of cases, one of the first surgeons to draw attention to the operation in England being the late Mr. Keetley.

It forms a satisfactory and safe method of enabling the whole colon to be irrigated with any desired solution, and at the same time does not leave the patient with an offensive and leaking opening.

As originally performed by Weir, the operation consisted of bringing the end of the appendix out of a wound in the abdomen and stitching it to the skin. The cæcum was not drawn up to the abdominal wall, and consequently it was possible for a loop of intestine to become strangulated around it and also, if inflammation of the appendix should occur, the peritoneal cavity might become infected. These objections, however, were soon realized and the cæcum pulled up so that the entire appendix lay in the thickness of the abdominal wall.

The operation is performed as follows : An oblique incision is made over McBurney's point in the same way as in the ordinary operation for appendicectomy. The incision need only be a short one, and an inch and a half is often sufficient. The peritoneal

APPENDICOSTOMY

cavity is opened and the appendix found. The meso-appendix is then divided close to the appendix for from $\frac{1}{2}$ to 1 inch, depending upon the length of the appendix; but in any case care should be taken not to sever the artery of the appendix. If it is cut, there is risk of the appendix sloughing through lack of adequate blood-supply. The artery should be looked for, and the meso-appendix only divided up to it, and no farther. The appendix is then brought out of the wound and pulled up until the cæcal wall comes well up against the parietal peritoneum. One or two catgut sutures may be inserted, so as to anchor the cæcal wall to the fascia and parietal peritoneum. Two or three stitches will then suffice to close the remainder of the wound. Lastly, a single stitch should be passed through the wall of the appendix, so that it can be anchored to the skin and prevented

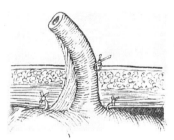

Fig. 75.—Diagram to show the method of fixing the cæcum and appendix to the abdominal wall.

from retracting. The dressings are then applied and the operation is finished. In applying the dressings, a roll of gauze should be placed on each side of the appendix to prevent the blood-supply being damaged by the pressure of the bandage.

If there is any doubt about the patency of the appendix, it should be opened at once, but if it is large and healthy it may be left, and opened two or three days later.

In performing the operation, and especially in closing the wound, the importance of preserving the blood-supply of the appendix should be borne in mind.

About two or three days later the dressings should be removed, and the appendix cut off about $\frac{1}{4}$ to $\frac{1}{2}$ an inch from the skin. It is better not to cut it flush with the skin. An appendicostomy catheter (No. 7 or No. 10) can then be passed into the cæcum through the stump of the appendix, and irrigation commenced. Later, any mucous membrane that projects above the skin level can be cut away so as to leave a neat opening.

The above seems to be the best procedure in view of leaving as good an opening as possible.

If the appendix is cut off at or soon after the operation, a certain amount of superficial suppuration in the wound will probably occur, and this often leads to some stricture at the orifice. The catheter should only be inserted in the canal for irrigation. If it is left in and happens to be rather a tight fit, the whole appendix may slough, owing to its presence interfering with the blood-supply, which, as the appendix is a vestigial organ, is often none too good.

Tuttle advises that at the end of thirty-six hours a catheter should be passed into the cæcum, and a ligature tied tightly round the appendix on to the catheter and left in position till it has amputated the appendix. As has already been mentioned,

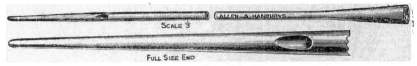

Fig. 76.—Appendicostomy catheter.

however, the continued presence of the catheter is liable to cause sloughing of the stump.

The operation can be performed in a very short time, and with the minimum of exposure of the abdominal cavity. It is practically free from any serious risk, and can be performed on patients whose general condition is bad and would contraindicate any more serious operation.

For these reasons it is admirably suited to such cases as ulcerative colitis and other suitable forms of colitis. The results obtained from irrigation of the colon through an appendicostomy wound are fully considered under the headings of the diseases for which it has been recommended.

It may happen that at the operation the appendix is found to be diseased, deformed, or rudimentary: in such cases considerable modification of the technique will be necessary to deal with it, or it may not be possible to utilize the appendix at all. Under such circumstances it should be removed, and some form of valvular cæcostomy, such as is presently described, performed.

It may be well to mention here that care should be taken as to the fluid used for irrigation. Considerable absorption occurs in the colon, and it is dangerous to put any fluid or dose of a drug into the colon that cannot safely be put into the stomach. This has not sometimes been sufficiently realized, and I have seen two cases of boracic acid poisoning, with a rash and vomiting, result from the use of boracic acid lotion for irrigation, and one case of carbolic acid poisoning from the use of weak lysol solution.

I have been able to collect 50 cases in which this operation has been performed, of which nine are my own. A careful analysis of these shows that while the operation is practically devoid of any risk as regards life, there are several minor complications which may result and cause trouble, though, as I shall be able to show, these may be avoided by care in performing the operation.

Six of the patients died, but in no instance was death attributable in any way to the operation. Two died, some months later, of cancer of the colon present at the time of operation. One died of peritonitis—the operation having been done to relieve distention; one died of miliary tuberculosis some weeks later; one of ulcerative colitis, for the relief of which the operation had been performed, and it was discovered post mortem that the ileum was also ulcerated; and one died from another operation performed some time later.

Minor complications occurred in nine cases. In one, the opening could not be kept open more than four weeks. In six cases the appendix sloughed: in four of these it was due to a catheter being left in the appendix; in the other two it was apparently due to the blood-supply having been damaged at the operation. In two of the cases in which the appendix sloughed, the opening became obliterated; but in the other three it was kept open by means of a rubber plug, and a useful opening resulted.

In two cases in which the appendix was cut off at the operation, the stump retracted inside the wound, resulting in suppuration and subsequent difficulty in inserting the catheter. In another case also, suppuration of the wound occurred, apparently from the same cause. In three cases the appendix at the operation was found to be diseased and its lumen obliterated. In each

298　　　APPENDICOSTOMY

of these a catheter was passed into the cæcum through a small opening, and part of it was then buried in the cæcal wall with Lembert sutures, the other end being brought out through the abdominal wall.

In one of my cases the appendix was found to be only an inch long and quite rudimentary, having a patent lumen for only half an inch from the cæcum. The patient was a stout woman with an abdominal wall four inches thick. The cæcum was stitched to the parietal peritoneum, and the end of the appendix cut off. A catheter was then passed through the short stump into the cæcum, and a ligature tied tightly round the stump on to the catheter, the other end of the catheter being brought out of the abdomen (see *Fig.* 77).

This case did very well, but the catheter or a solid rubber

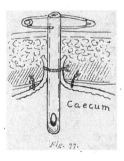

Fig. 77.

plug has to be left in the canal to prevent its closing, as the walls consist only of fibrous tissue. In another case, I had to adopt the same procedure because the appendix had no lumen for three-quarters of its extent.

In only one case was there any leakage of fæcal material. The patient was a woman, and the operation had been performed for chronic colitis. There was considerable leakage from the opening. On enquiry I found that the surgeon who performed the operation divided the whole of the meso-appendix, and in consequence the entire appendix sloughed and came away. The result was therefore, in reality, a fæcal fistula communicating with the cæcum, and not an appendicostomy opening.

The results of appendicostomy as regards the operation itself are most satisfactory. After the wound has healed the opening

APPENDICOSTOMY

is barely noticeable, appearing merely as a small pink spot on the abdominal wall (see *Fig.* 78). No leakage at all occurs through the opening when the catheter is withdrawn, or at least has not in any of the cases I have seen. In one, I injected sufficient water into the colon to cause marked distention of the abdomen, and on removing the catheter there was no leakage from the opening. Neither flatus nor fæces escape, and the presence of the opening causes the patient no inconvenience whatever. Most patients find it quite unnecessary to wear anything over it.

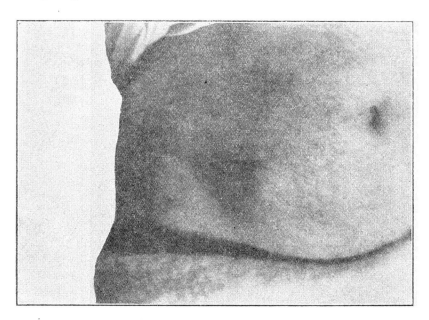

Fig. 78.—Photograph showing the appearance of an appendicostomy opening three years after operation. The opening is still patent. (*Author's case.*)

Should it be necessary to close the opening, all that is required is a touch with the cautery or the application of a little nitric acid to the mucous lining of the opening, the wound readily healing in a few days.

It is better to keep it open till all possibility of its being required is gone, and as it causes no inconvenience, this can readily be done.

300 CÆCOSTOMY FOR IRRIGATION

Irrigation through the opening can be carried out easily by the patient, and he is not prevented from living his usual life or from going into the society of others in any way. Several patients assured me that the opening caused no inconvenience, and one (a labouring man) said that he found it saved him time, as he was always certain of being able to empty his bowel in three or four minutes.

All that is necessary to irrigate the bowel is to pass a catheter into the opening and attach a Higginson's syringe to the other

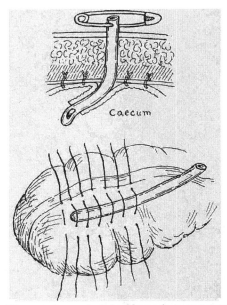

Fig. 79.—Diagram to show method of making a valvular cæcostomy in cases where the appendix cannot be utilized.

end. The fluid is then pumped into the cæcum in a few minutes, and allowed to run out at the anus. If oil is used it is best put in with a glass syringe, as it flows too slowly through a funnel.

CÆCOSTOMY FOR IRRIGATION OF THE COLON.

In cases where the appendix cannot be used, this operation, or some modification of it, can be performed.

A small opening is made in the wall of the cæcum just large

enough to admit the end of a No. 10 catheter (of soft rubber). The end of the catheter is passed through this hole for about ¾ inch. A series of Lembert sutures are then commenced, well beyond the hole, and continued over the catheter for about 1½ inches. These should be so placed that, when they are tied up, the catheter for about an inch will be buried in the wall of the cæcum. The cæcal wall where the catheter passes through is then anchored firmly to the bottom of the wound, the base of the catheter is brought out of the wound, and the remainder closed.

This makes a very good opening and does not leak, but it is necessary for a small rubber plug to be worn to prevent the opening from cicatrizing up.

Chapter XXII.

RESECTION AND ANASTOMOSIS OF THE COLON.

THE PREPARATION OF THE PATIENT FOR AN OPERATION UPON THE COLON.

ONE of the most important factors in obtaining successful results from operations upon the colon is the preparation of the patient. When we have to operate for acute obstruction, or other urgent symptoms due to disease in the colon, it is often impossible to have the patient properly prepared. Under such circumstances immediate operation is of more importance than any other factor, and the advantages which will result from careful preparation have to be sacrificed. For this reason, most operations performed for urgent obstructive symptoms are of a simple nature, usually some form of colotomy. In most cases in which an anastomosis or resection has to be performed there is no great urgency, and careful preparation of the patient is possible.

This is of almost as much importance as the skill of the operator; and the best results are undoubtedly obtained by surgeons who pay most attention to this part of the treatment. It is not sufficient for the preparation to be left to the nurse, with a few brief directions; the surgeon should himself see that the preparatory treatment is carefully and efficiently carried out. A week, or even longer, is not too much to devote to getting the patient ready for operation if an anastomosis is to be performed. There are two objects to be aimed at: first, that the colon shall at the time of operation be as nearly as possible empty; and second, that its contents shall be rendered as far as possible aseptic. It is, of course, not possible to render the interior of the colon aseptic, but much may be done to rid it of pathogenic bacteria, and to lower the virulence of those that remain.

The bowel should first of all be well cleared by means of a purge, and for this purpose nothing is better than a dose of castor oil (from a half to one ounce). This may with advantage be given a week before the operation. After this, the bowels should be kept acting daily by some mild aperient, such as a small dose of magnesia or cascara. The patient should not be restricted as regards his diet, but be instructed to eat only plain cooked food, and to avoid vegetables, fruit, or other substances which will leave an indigestible residue. The teeth should be examined, and if carious or otherwise unhealthy, the patient should go to a dentist and have them put right or extracted. An antiseptic mouth-wash should in any case be ordered twice daily to ensure that the mouth is as clean as possible.

There are several ways in which we can advantageously modify the number and variety of the bacteria in the colon. We can give intestinal antiseptics by the mouth, such as liquor hydrarg. perchlor. ʒj, salol gr. x, or beta-naphthol gr. x, three times daily. A more recent and more efficient method of purifying the colon is by the use of the lactic acid ferment. This acts by introducing into the intestine a harmless micro-organism which will destroy and take the place of those which are already present. The best preparation for the purpose is a fresh culture of the Bulgarian bacillus prepared in a scientific laboratory. Two tablets of the dried culture should be given three times a day in a little sweetened milk. If a fresh laboratory culture is unobtainable, a good brand of soured milk should be given, the dose being about two pints a day. In either case it should be given before meals, and at the end of a day or two the stools should be examined for the bacillus. As soon as the bacillus has appeared in the stools, the dose by the mouth may be cut down by a third. This treatment must be commenced some time before the operation, in order to give the bacillus time to become acclimatized to the intestine. Occasionally some degree of digestive disturbance follows the use of the lactic acid bacillus, and in that case the operation should not be performed until it has passed off. The effect of this treatment will be to render the colon as nearly aseptic as it is possible to make it..

On the day before the operation the patient should be given a smart purge, and the diet be reduced to a light and easily digestible form. On the evening before the operation a soap-and-water enema (two pints) should be given. I always order 15 gr. of pulv. ipecac. comp. or 1 oz. of mist. catechu comp. to be given at the same time as the enema. Next day, four hours before the operation, an enema of plain warm water (two pints) should be given. The object of the opium is to arrest peristalsis and to prevent the last enema from inducing peristaltic contractions, as it otherwise will do, and so bringing down more material into the colon. It also has the advantage of helping the patient to sleep the night before the operation, which he will often be unable to do without aid. Whatever opinions surgeons may hold with regard to the use of opium after abdominal operations, there can be no objection to its employment beforehand.

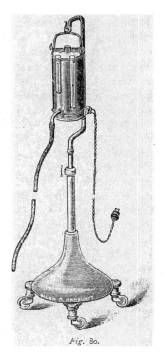

Fig. 80.

The patient's abdomen will, of course, be shaved, and a compress applied on the day previous to operation. No food should be given on the morning of the operation, though a cup of weak tea or some other form of fluid may be allowed two or three hours before the time. An exception to this, however, is often advisable in the case of elderly and very young patients. In addition to the above preparatory treatment, I usually give

PREPARATION OF PATIENT

the patient two or three teaspoonfuls of white vaseline by the mouth for two days before the operation, and continue it afterwards. This makes certain that the fæces will not become consolidated, and that there can only be liquid fæces to pass the line of anastomosis. Petroleum may either be given as white vaseline, to which some flavouring has been added, such as peppermint, or as the liquid petroleum of the Pharmacopœia.

If it is anticipated that the operation will cause shock, I like to give a hypodermic injection of morphia, gr. $\frac{1}{4}$, just before commencing the anæsthetic. This also reduces the amount of anæsthetic required, and renders subsequent vomiting less likely to occur. The patient should be well protected against cold and exposure during the operation, either by a jacket and trousers of gamgee tissue, or by some form of woollen clothing which will not require to be removed.

Mr. Arbuthnot Lane's plan for preventing shock in these operations by the subcutaneous infusion of warm saline during and after the operation is excellent. *Fig.* 80 shows a very useful apparatus, by means of which the saline can be kept at the desired temperature for long periods without constant attention. All that is necessary is to connect the apparatus to a large hypodermic needle put under the skin of the axilla, and to keep the tank filled with sterilized salt solution. The tank should only be raised about a foot above the needle, so that infusion occurs slowly. The heat is maintained at the required temperature by electricity from the ordinary house supply.

RESECTION OF THE COLON.

The colon may be resected in part or in whole. The best and easiest method of dealing with a seriously diseased colon is to resect a length containing the diseased area. If the entire colon is so seriously diseased that it is not capable of recovery; it can be completely resected.

Whenever possible, that portion which it is proposed to resect should be drawn out of the abdomen, and the abdominal wound and peritoneum carefully protected by gauze packing. The loop of bowel is then, as far as possible, emptied by milking out the contents, and an intestinal clamp is placed on the bowel-wall above and below the points at which it is proposed to divide the gut. The division should always be made through healthy bowel-wall, and well clear of the lesion. In the case of cancer, the bowel should be divided at least one clear inch from the edges of the growth. In order to be certain of preserving a good blood-supply to the edges of the bowel, the bowel-wall should be divided slightly obliquely, the greatest amount of bowel being removed on the side opposite the mesocolon (see Fig. 81). When the bowel has been divided, and the diseased area removed, the ends of the divided gut should be cleaned with gauze to remove any fæcal material. The mucous membrane always prolapses to some extent beyond the other coats, and if anastomosis is to be performed, this projecting ring of mucosa should be carefully trimmed off with scissors, so that all the coats are left level. This materially aids accurate apposition of the ends when performing anastomosis.

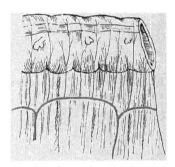

Fig. 81.—Diagram to show the way in which the arteries pass from the arterial arcades to the colon wall.

Method of Dealing with the Mesocolon.—If resection has been performed for malignant disease, a wedge-shaped portion of the mesocolon should always be removed in one piece with the resected bowel. And it is advisable to remove as far as possible all the lymphatic area immediately draining the growth. The indications for removing this area have been already discussed fully in Chapter XVIII.

When it is not necessary to remove any of the mesocolon, the loose fold left after resection can be turned back on itself and sutured together. All that is necessary is to ensure that no opening or pocket is left which might result in the formation of an internal hernia at a later period.

There are various methods of dealing with the bowel after resection, and these, and the indications for each, have been

ANASTOMOSIS

already discussed. It remains to describe the various methods of anastomosis.

ANASTOMOSIS.

I shall only describe anastomosis by direct suture, for although there are a great variety of methods depending upon the use of some special apparatus, such as a bobbin or button, these have now been almost entirely discarded in favour of direct suture. This is both better and safer than the use of bobbins, and can be performed as quickly after a little practice. Many successful anastomoses have been performed in the colon with a Murphy's button; but on the other hand there have been many fatalities which were directly attributable to its use.

End-to-end Anastomosis.—This is as a rule only possible in the transverse and pelvic portions of the colon. The results of end-to-end anastomosis are not nearly so satisfactory as in the case of the small intestine. In the latter the operation has quite a low death-rate; but in the colon the mortality is nearly 30 per cent.

Out of 89 cases of which I have been able to find records, 60 recovered and 29 died. Moreover, of those patients who recovered, a number developed a fæcal fistula as the result of the operation.

End-to-end Anastomosis by Suture.—The colon having been clamped and the diseased portion resected, the two ends of the colon enclosed in the clamps are brought together, so that they lie parallel with one another. The mucous membrane which generally projects from each end of the bowel is then cut off with scissors, so that the mucous membrane is flush with the other bowel coats; this is advisable, as it enables a much better union to be made. A single mattress suture is next put in, taking up all the coats and joining the two mesenteric borders of the colon. This suture should bring the two mesenteric borders into accurate apposition, and the knot should be tied on the mucous side; the ends should be left long to act as a guide while the remaining sutures are being passed.

A continuous through-and-through suture, taking up all the coats, should next be inserted, starting from the mesenteric border and continued halfway round the bowel. It should then be tied off, and a similar suture started also from the mesenteric border and carried along the opposite side. After the first turn of this suture has been inserted, the guide suture in the mesenteric border should be cut off. The two continuous sutures are tied together where they meet opposite the mesenteric attachment.

Over this first suture line a second suture of fine silk should now be inserted uniting the peritoneal coats only. This peritoneal suture should preferably be inserted in two portions, each going halfway round the bowel; this minimizes the risk of puckering the bowel.

Some surgeons prefer to use silk for the first suture which passes through the mucous membrane, but stout chromicized

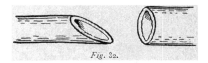

Fig. 82.

catgut is perhaps better, for this suture must come out, as it becomes infected from the mucous membrane, and if made of silk, a certain amount of sloughing will accompany its discharge into the bowel. In one instance I examined with the sigmoidoscope the line of union two months after end-to-end anastomosis had been performed in the sigmoid flexure, and was able to see the small ulcers in the mucous membrane all round the bowel where the silk stitch had been, and which were still unhealed.

After the ends of the bowel have been joined, the mesosigmoid or mesentery should be repaired so as not to leave a hole through

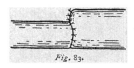

Fig. 83.

which small bowel may become strangulated. This is easily managed with a continuous catgut or silk suture.

In the case of resection of the cæcal end of the colon, if the ileum and colon are to be united end to end, it is necessary first of all to make the two ends of bowel the same size. There are several methods of doing this.

The ileum may be cut obliquely and the colon transversely. (See *Fig.* 82).

The ileum may be joined to the colon and then the excess of colon sewn up. (See *Fig.* 83).

ANASTOMOSIS

A V-shaped piece of the colon may be cut out on the side opposite the mesenteric attachment, and the V-shaped wound sewn up to make the end of the colon the same size as the ileum. This is Madelung's method. (See *Fig.* 84.)

Doyen has invented an ingenious method by which a sort of artificial ileocæcal valve is formed. The end of the ileum is turned inside out so as to form a cuff. The end of the colon is

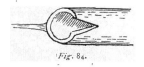

Fig. 84.

next reduced till it is the same size as the ileum, the ileum is inserted into it, and the edge of the turned-back cuff sewn to the edge of the colon. (See *Fig.* 85.)

Lateral Anastomosis.—Lateral, instead of end-to-end anastomosis, may be performed after resection of the colon or in performing a short-circuiting operation. When the ileum and colon have to be joined it is an easier operation than end-to-end

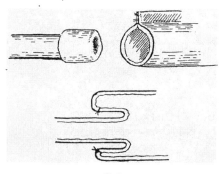

Fig 85.

anastomosis. If performed after resection, the two ends of the bowel are first closed. This may be done by sewing up the end and invaginating it, a purse-string suture or a series of Lembert sutures being afterwards inserted to further protect the end. Mr. Lane's method is to put a ligature round the ends of the divided bowel and then invaginate the ligatured end with a purse-string suture.

ANASTOMOSIS

.The two portions of bowel which are to be united are then placed side by side—care being taken to see that peristalsis will occur in the right direction—and joined together side to side for about 2 to 2½ inches with a peritoneal stitch taking up the peritoneal and muscular coats only. This suture is not cut, but left long.

An incision in the long axis of the bowel is now made into both portions of bowel, about 2 inches long and close to the line of suture. Any projecting mucous membrane is cut away, and a continuous catgut suture is inserted, taking up all the bowel coats. This is continued right round the openings until they are joined together. Lastly, the peritoneal stitch is continued until it reaches the place where it started, thus forming a double line of suture and covering in the first line.

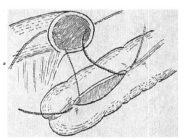

Fig. 86.—Diagram to show the method of inserting guide sutures in performing anastomosis by implantation.

When possible it is better to perform the anastomosis before the resection, and also to close the ends of the portion of colon which it is proposed to resect. There is thus considerably less danger of soiling the peritoneum.

In any case, after performing the anastomosis, the edges of the divided mesocolon must be carefully stitched together to avoid leaving any gap or hole through which the small bowel can pass and become strangulated.

Lateral Implantation.—This is in some ways preferable to lateral anastomosis, and is favoured by many surgeons. It is much better than end-to-end anastomosis when dealing with the ileum and colon, as it removes the difficulty of the different sizes of the two portions of bowel. If performed after resection, the end of the colon is first stitched up, then an incision of suitable length is made into the side of the blind end of the colon, and about one to two inches from the end in the long axis of the bowel. A guide suture is then inserted taking up the end of this incision and the middle of the side wall of the ileum, a similar suture being placed on the other side. These ensure the ends of the bowel being stitched together correctly, and are useful in holding the bowel edges in position during suturing. The two edges are then sutured together, taking up all the coats, and last of all a protecting peritoneal line of suture is put in over the first, and the mesentery is stitched together. (See *Fig.* 86.)

Charters Symonds advises using a Murphy's button for lateral implantation. The slight saving of time obtained by this method, however, seems insufficient to compensate for the increased risk of introducing a foreign body into the colon.

Ileo-sigmoidostomy.—This may be done either by lateral anastomosis or by implantation of the ileum into the sigmoid flexure. Lane, who has been one of the chief advocates of ileo-sigmoidostomy, advises division of the ileum about 6 inches from the ileocæcal valve, and implantation of the proximal end into the sigmoid flexure by suture. The distal end of the ileum is closed.

If the patient is so ill as to render a short operation of paramount importance, a Murphy's button may be used to form the junction between the ileum and pelvic colon ; but in skilled hands there is little, if any, saving of time to be secured by this method. It is important to carefully stitch together the mesocolon and the divided edge of the mesentery, in order to ensure that no gap is left through which subsequent strangulation might occur.

Shortening of the Mesosigmoid.—This operation may be done to prevent the recurrence of a volvulus, and to prevent acute flexures from occurring and causing obstruction or chronic constipation. It may be performed in cases where there is an abnormally long mesosigmoid, and is attended with less risk than the alternative operation of resection of the elongated loop.

A series of Lembert sutures are inserted in the long axis of the mesocolon, and parallel with one another. The sutures should all be inserted on one side of the mesentery only, preferably on the outer side, and should take up the peritoneum only, special care being taken to avoid wounding the veins when inserting the sutures. The first row is tied up, then a second row is inserted over these, and so on, until the mesocolon has been sufficiently shortened. As a rule, it is found, after all the sutures have been tied, that a kink has been produced in the colon at either end of the line of sutures. To remedy this, a few more Lembert sutures should be inserted opposite the kinks in such a way as to straighten them out. (See *Fig.* 32, p. 91.)

Colopexy.—This operation is sometimes performed to prevent the reformation of a volvulus, or to cure an abnormal kink or angle in the colon which is causing chronic obstruction. It has also been done in some cases of visceroptosis, and to cure prolapse.

The part of the colon which requires anchoring is usually the sigmoid flexure. The bowel is fixed by a series of sutures either to the walls of the iliac fossa, or in some cases to the abdominal wall. When the portion of the bowel has been selected which it is proposed to fix, the peritoneum should be scraped or in part removed, and a corresponding portion of peritoneum removed from that portion of the abdominal wall or iliac fossa to which it is proposed to attach it. It is better to select, if possible, the iliac fossa, as this is fixed, whereas the abdominal wall is constantly moving. The selected and prepared portion of colon is next secured to its prepared bed by sutures. These sutures must be very carefully inserted with fine peritoneal needles, care being taken not to perforate the bowel-wall, but at the same time to obtain a good hold. It is also necessary to see that the blood-supply is not interfered with, or the bowel kinked.

Colopexy does not appear to be very satisfactory, as in several instances in which it has been performed to prevent the reformation of a volvulus it has failed, and at a subsequent operation the bowel has been found free and with no trace of the previous fixation.

METHODS OF RESTORING THE BOWEL AFTER RESECTION OF GROWTHS JUST ABOVE THE RECTO-SIGMOIDAL JUNCTION.

It often happens, after resecting a growth at the lower end of the pelvic colon, that it is not possible to deal with the ends of the bowel by any of the ordinary methods. The lower stump is too short to reach the skin, and owing to its immobility, and position at the back of the pelvis, it is impossible to perform anastomosis, although the upper stump of colon is quite long enough to reach it.

AFTER RESECTION OF GROWTHS

There are two methods by which the bowel can be restored under such circumstances. If the upper stump is long and has a long mesentery (not less than 5 inches), the surgeon can free the lower stump all round from the abdomen, and, by making

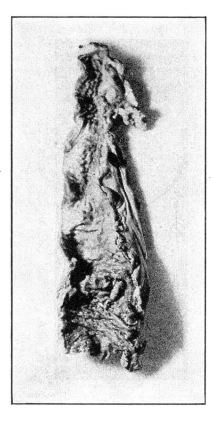

Fig. 87.—Photograph of the parts removed by abdomino-perineal excision for cancer at the recto-sigmoidal junction. The specimen includes the whole rectum and half the sigmoid flexure. It measured 14 inches in length. The patient made a good recovery, and had excellent control over the new rectum, which was formed by bringing down the stump of the sigmoid flexure and stitching it to the anus. (*Author's case*).

an incision in the perineum, excise the entire lower portion of bowel, in fact, perform abdomino-perineal excision of the rectum, bringing the stump of the sigmoid down to the anus and fixing it there. This is a formidable operation, but, if successful, it gives very good results. A photograph is appended (*Fig.* 87) showing the parts removed in such a case. The patient recovered and had excellent control over the bowel.

Another method of dealing with such cases, and one which is simpler and does not involve the removal of a normal rectum, is as follows :—After the growth has been resected, a long glass tube or one of the author's rubber tubes is tied into the upper stump of the pelvic colon, and the free end of this tube is then passed into the lower stump and pushed down until it can be drawn out of the anus by an assistant. The edges of the lower stump are made to invaginate, so that the peritoneal surfaces of the two portions of bowel come into contact. A few sutures are then inserted, if possible, to fix the two portions of bowel together, and the abdominal wound is closed. The line of junction cannot leak until the tube separates, and by that time firm union should have taken place. (See *Fig.* 88.)

The condition produced is practically a short artificial intussusception, the two peritoneal coats being in apposition, and the ends of the mucous coats close together, though not necessarily touching each other. Owing to the glass tube tied into the upper portion of the bowel, no leakage can occur, and the ends of the bowel have about a week in which to become united to each other before there is any possibility of strain being thrown upon the line of union ; while the tube is still in position the bowels can be freely opened without any risk of leakage, and this is a very great advantage in the case of an anastomosis so near the rectum.

The following is an instance in which this operation was performed with successful results :—

Case.—I saw the patient, a man, aged 53 years, on Oct. 18th, 1907, on account of hæmorrhage from the bowel. His history was that for nearly twelve months he had been passing mucus and occasionally blood, and had had attacks of pain in the abdomen. About a month previously he had a profuse hæmorrhage from the bowel, and this had occurred again the day before I saw him, and had been accompanied by severe pain in the abdomen lasting for about half an hour. On examination per rectum nothing abnormal could be felt, but very high up a large resisting mass could be felt through the anterior rectal wall. Under ether, by bimanual examination, and after stretching the sphincters so as to allow of two fingers being inserted into the rectum, a growth could be distinctly felt in

AFTER RESECTION OF GROWTHS 315

the lower part of the sigmoid flexure. This diagnosis was confirmed by sigmoidoscopy.

The operation was performed on Nov. 4th. The patient was anæsthetized with ether by the open method. The patient having been placed in the Trendelenburg position, an incision was made through the outer part of the rectus sheath on the left side of the abdomen and extending right down to the pubes. On opening the abdomen I found that the lower part of the growth extended down to within one and a half inches of the recto-sigmoidal junction, and that a loop of the sigmoid flexure above the growth had become adherent to, and was involved in, it. This necessitated the removal of all but a few inches of the sigmoid flexure if the growth was to be removed. The sigmoid flexure was divided above the involved

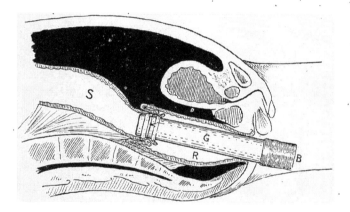

Fig. 88.—(S) Sigmoid. (R) Rectum. (G) Glass tube, to the upper end of which the sigmoid is tied. (B) Piece of rubber tube to prevent glass tube from slipping up into rectum.

loop, and the mesosigmoid was stripped up from the posterior pelvic wall and the vessels clamped as they were divided. This procedure was rendered necessary by the fact that some of the glands in the mesosigmoid were involved. As a result of the stripping up of the peritoneum, the great iliac vessels were laid bare. The sigmoid flexure at the recto-sigmoidal junction was now divided an inch below the growth, and the adherent loops were removed. The peritoneum was brought together by stitches over the posterior pelvic wall, and all bleeding points were ligated. At this stage, owing to the rectum not having been properly emptied previously to the operation, some soiling of the pelvic peritoneum unfortunately took place. Any of the ordinary methods of end-to-end anastomosis were quite impossible owing to the depth of the wound and to the fact that there was no stump of bowel below, but merely a hole in the pelvic floor. I tied a glass Keith's tube into the upper end of the sigmoid flexure, and passed the free end of this tube, to which a piece of large-bore rubber tubing had previously been attached, down into the rectum from the abdominal cavity. An assistant then caught this with forceps introduced per anum, and drew it out of the anus. By drawing on the Keith's tube, the upper end of the sigmoid flexure was invaginated into the upper end of the rectum, thus forming a kind of intussusception. Two or three silk stitches were then put in to prevent the invagination from coming undone. A drainage-tube was then inserted and the abdominal wound was closed in separate layers.

The bowels were freely opened with calomel on the third day through the tube. The tube separated and came away on the seventh day; after this a fæcal fistula formed along the track of the drainage tube, and there was some discharge for a time, but the bowels continued to act by the rectum. The patient made a good recovery without any bad symptoms, and although the fæcal fistula was a troublesome complication, it soon began to close, and in the course of a couple of weeks only allowed a little flatus to escape occasionally and soon healed.

The patient is quite well at the present time, two years after operation. There is no trace of a stricture, and he has normal control over the action of his bowels.

Resection of the Entire Colon.—I believe the first case in which this operation was performed successfully was one in which Lienthall, an American surgeon, resected the whole colon for multiple adenomata. The operation was performed on June 15th, 1900. The patient was a woman, aged 21, whose colon from end to end was covered internally with small adenomata which caused dangerous and intractable hæmorrhage. The operation was performed in two stages, and the patient recovered. Arbuthnot Lane was, however, the first to complete the resection at one operation. He has performed it a considerable number of times, and has proved that it can be done with a comparatively low mortality.

The technique is as follows :—A large median incision having been made, and the abdomen opened, the ileum is divided at a point about five or six inches from the cæcum. A ligature is first placed round the ileum, and the latter is then divided with a cautery. The stump is next buried in the proximal bowel by means of a purse-string suture. Next, the adhesions and peritoneum which bind the cæcum and ascending colon to the

AFTER RESECTION OF GROWTHS

posterior abdominal wall are divided, and the bowel is raised until the vessels supplying it are exposed. These are seized in forceps and ligatured. The transverse colon is similarly treated. The vessels are first controlled, and then the colon is freed. The descending colon, and as much as is considered advisable of the sigmoid flexure, are similarly freed. A point having been chosen in the sigmoid, which will leave a long enough stump after division to enable the anastomosis to be performed, the bowel is divided at this spot, the lower end being closed in the same way as in dealing with the ileum. The whole colon is now free and can be removed. The closed end of the ileum and the closed stump of the sigmoid are then brought together and joined by lateral anastomosis. Lastly, the edge of the mesentery of the ileum is stitched to the edge of the mesosigmoid, so as to prevent there being any gap through which bowel might prolapse and become strangulated. Mr. Lane passes a fine gut ligature through the free incised margin of the mesentery of the ileum, and then beneath the peritoneum forming the outer wall of the mesorectum. When this is tied it brings the rectum to the middle line of the pelvis and fixes it in that situation. The operation may also be performed in two stages, by first doing an ileo-sigmoidostomy, and later resecting the colon.

INDEX

	PAGE
ABDOMEN, palpation of the	43
Abdominal muscles, exercises for strengthening the	224
Abnormalities, congenital	58
Abscess, as complication of ulcerative colitis	178
— a result of pericolitis	193, 198
Absorption of food constituents by the colon	14
Acute dilatation	32
Adeno-carcinoma	249
Adenomata, multiple	237
— villous	237
Adhesions following pericolitis	194
— a cause of constipation	95, 221
— and kinking	92
— — — symptoms	94
— — — treatment	102
Age incidence in volvulus	87
Amœbic dysentery	156
Anæsthetic, examination under	55
Anastomosis, spontaneous, from cancer of colon	260
— technique of	29, 307
Anatomy and development	1
Animals, variations of the colon in	1
Antiperistalsis	20
Anus, artificial, closure by operation	291
— — operation to form	280
Appendices epiploicæ causing constriction	98
Appendicitis a cause of kinking	98
— causing mucous colitis	135
Appendicostomy for chronic colitis	145
— catheter	296
— for constipation	227
—.— dilated colon	74
— — hæmorrhagic colitis	169
— opening, to close	299
— technique of	294
— in tuberculosis	214
— — ulcerative colitis	174
Arsenic in chronic colitis	141
Arterial circulation	4
— thrombosis a cause of meteorism	32
Arteries, embolism of colic	235
Artificial anus, closure by operation	291
— — operation to form	280

	PAGE
Artificial anus, physiological results of	29
— — in ulcerative colitis	174
Asylum dysentery	156
BACILLUS bulgaricus	38
— — in preparing patient for operation	303
— coli	38
— dysenteriæ	154
— of tubercle	40
Bacteria in colon, modification in preparing for operation	303
Bacteriology of the colon	37
— — ulcerative colitis	156
Bailey's modification of Witzel's colotomy	283
Belladonna in chronic colitis	141
— — enterospasm	153
Bismuth in X-ray diagnosis	51
Blood in stools, diagnostic importance of	57
Blood-supply, interference with, a cause of meteorism	32
Blood-vessels	4
Bougies and tubes in diagnosis	55
Bulgarian bacillus	38
— — in preparing patient for operation	303
CÆCOSTOMY for chronic colitis	144
— — irrigation of colon	300
— technique of	289
— for ulcerative colitis	174
Cæcum as an organ of digestion	1
— volvulus of	83
Cancer	249
— associated with pericolitis	195
— a cause of chronic mucous colitis	136
— — — intussusception	120
— indications for removing	267
— lines of extension of growth	253
— morbid anatomy	250
— palliative operations	273
— predisposing causes	250
— recurrence after excision	272
— secondary results of	260
— spontaneous anastomosis in	261
— symptoms	255
— treatment	263

INDEX 319.

	PAGE
Carbon dioxide, its origin in acute dilatation	33
Catarrhal colitis causing mucous colitis	137
Cholin in the fæces	26
Chronic constipation	218
—— treatment	221
—— mucous or membranous colitis	127
Closure of fæcal fistula by operation	290
CO_2, its origin in acute dilatation	33
Colectomy, physiological results of	28
Colica mucosa	127
Colitis, caused by adhesions	95
— chronic mucous or membranous	24, 127
— — — operations for	143
— — — pathology and etiology	132
— — — treatment	139
— — — symptoms	128
— hæmorrhagic	167
— polyposa	237
— tuberculous	201
— ulcerative	154
— — bacteriology	156
— — etiology	155
— — pathology	157
— — prognosis	165
— — symptoms	161
— — treatment	172
— various types of inflammation in	137
Colon, length of	2
— surface markings of	8
Colopexy, technique of	312
Colostomy for ulcerative colitis	174
Colotomy	280
— in cancer	264
— closure of	290
— for chronic colitis	144
— — congenital dilatation and hypertrophy	73
— inguinal, technique of	281
— lumbar, technique of	285
— opening, control over	286
— as palliative in cancer	275
— Paul's method	287
— preparation of patient for	302
— sensation at the opening after	15
— valvular	283
Congenital abnormalities of the colon	58
— — peritoneum or mesentery	59
— causes of volvulus	78
— dilatation and hypertrophy	61
— — — diagnosis of	64
— — — etiology of	65
— — — morbid anatomy of	68
— — — prognosis of	72
— — — treatment of	72
Constipation, adhesions a cause of	93

	PAGE
Constipation, atonic	220
— in cancer	258
— chronic	218
— — operative treatment	226
— — treatment	221
— exercises for	224
— use of X rays in diagnosis of	218
Contents of the colon	24
Contractions of mesosigmoid from pericolitis	196
Croup, mucous	127
Deformities of mesosigmoid from pericolitis	196
Development of the Colon	9
Diagnosis by means of bougies and tubes	55
— methods of	41
— the sigmoidoscope in	44
— X rays in	51
Diarrhœa, causes of	26
— membranous or mucous	127
— in multiple polypi of the colon	243
— in ulcerative colitis	161
Diet in chronic colitis	141
— Von Noorden's	141
Dilatation, acute	32
— and hypertrophy, congenital	61
— post-operative, causes of	35
— resulting from cancer	261
— secondary results of	68
Distention or stercoral ulcers	169
Diverticula causing pericolitis	181
Doyen's method of anastomosis	309
Dysentery, bacillary, and ulcerative colitis	156
— stricture after	234
— tropical, and ulcerative colitis	154
Electrical treatment of adhesions	103
— — chronic constipation	225
Embolism of colic blood-vessels	235
End-to-end anastomosis, technique of	307
Enteritis membranacea	127
Entero-colitis	127
Enteroliths causing chronic constipation	228
Enteroptosis causing mucous colitis	135
— of transverse colon	107
Enterospasm	150
Enterotome for closing colotomy opening	292
Epicolic glands	7
Examination of the stools	56
Exercises for chronic constipation	224
Excision of bowel for cancer	263
— — — physiological results of	28
Exploratory laparotomy, when indicated	56

INDEX

	PAGE
FÆCAL calculi	228
— fistula, closure by operation	290
— impaction	228
— — symptoms	230
— — treatment	231
Fæces, acid reaction of	27
— bacteriological content of	37
— colour of	26
— examination of	56
— in mucous colitis	130
— normal and abnormal constituents in	24
Fat in the stools	25
Fibrolysin in treatment of adhesions	103
Fistula, fæcal, closure by operation	290
Fistulæ following pericolitis	194
Flexner's acid bacillus in ulcerative colitis	156
Fœtus, development of the colon in the	9
Follicular ulceration	166
Food constituents, absorption by the colon	14
— indigestible, a cause of intussusception	120
— time occupied in reaching and passing colon	19
Functions of the large intestine	13
GANGRENE causing intussusception	120
Gas-pipe colon	212
Glandular system	7
Glutinous diarrhœa	127
Granular colitis causing chronic mucous colitis	137
Growths in pelvic colon, restoring bowel after resection of	312
HÆMORRHAGE as complication of ulcerative colitis	178
Hæmorrhagic colitis	167
Hepatic flexure, cancer of	269
Hernia of the colon	111
Hirschsprung's disease	62
History as guide to diagnosis	41
Hydrotherapy in chronic constipation	226
Hyperplastic tuberculosis	202
Hypertrophic colitis with chronic mucous colitis	137
Hypertrophy and dilatation, congenital	61
Hyrax, arrangement of the cæcum in the	2
IDIOPATHIC dilatation	62
Iguana, function of cæcum in the	1
Ileocæcal angle, cancer of	255
— artery and its branches	5
— valve, anatomy of	3

	PAGE
Ileo-colostomy as palliative in cancer	274
Ileo-sigmoidostomy for chronic colitis	145
— for chronic constipation	228
— — dilated colon	75
— methods of	311
— — physiological results of	28
Indicanuria, Obermeyer's test for	57
Inflammation causing chronic mucous colitis	137
Inguinal colotomy	281
Injection treatment of intussusception	124
Injury to the colon in animals, sensory effect of	15
— — effect of experimental	15
Intestinal sand	25, 131
Intra-abdominal pressure, to restore	109
Intussusception	114
— etiology	115
— experimental	115
— pathology	120
— prognosis	126
— spontaneous elimination of	121
— symptoms	122
— treatment	124
Irrigation of colon, appendicostomy for	294
— — cæcostomy for	300
— — fluid used in	297
KINKING and adhesions	92
LACTIC acid bacilli	38
— — ferment in preparing patient for operation	303
Lane's method of anastomosis	309
Laparotomy, exploratory, when indicated	56
Lateral anastomosis, technique of	309
— implantation of bowel	310
Lemur, arrangement of the colon in the	2
Lienteric diarrhœa, causes of	26
Lumbar colotomy	285
Lymphatics	5
MADELUNG's method of anastomosis	309
Malformations giving rise to volvulus	78
Malignant disease	249
— — causing chronic mucous colitis	136
Massage for adhesions	102
— chronic constipation	223
Membranous colitis	127
Mental condition in mucous colitis	130

INDEX

	PAGE
Mesentery, abnormalities of, causing volvulus	78
— congenital abnormalities of	59
— development of the	11
Mesocolon, operation for shortening	92
— method of dealing with, in resection	306
Mesosigmoid, deformities and contractions following pericolitis	196
— operation for shortening the	311
Meteorism	32
— post-operative, causes of	35
Methods of diagnosis	41
— — restoring the bowel after resection of growths	312
Micro-organisms in intestinal contents	37
Monkeys, the cæcum in	1
Morbid physiology	28
Mucous or membranous colitis	127
— secretion and diarrhœa	26
Mucus, diagnostic importance of	56
— normal presence in colon	24, 56
Multiple polypi	237
Murphy's button in anastomosis	268, 307
NERVE supply	14
Nervous symptoms in mucous colitis	130
Neurin in the fæces	26
Neurosis theory of mucous colitis	132
Normal contents of the colon	24
Nothnagel's neurosis theory of mucous colitis	132
OBERMEYER's test for indicanuria	57
Obstruction due to cancer, treatment by operation	263
— chronic, from angulation or kinking	96
Occlusion of colon, physiological results of	28
Olive oil in chronic colitis	140
Omentum, development of the	11
Operation, preparation of patient for	302
Orang-utang, the cæcum in	1
PAIN in the colon only indirect	15
Palpation of the abdomen	43
Paracolic glands	7
Patient, preparation of, for operation	302
Paul's method of colotomy	287
— operation in cancer	265
Pelvic colon, anatomy of	9
— — volvulus of	83
Percussion of the abdomen	43
Perforating pericolitis, treatment	199
— ulcer, treatment	176

	PAGE
Perforation causing pericolitis	188
— of colic ulcer	160, 170
Pericolitis	179
— etiology	180
— diverticula causing	186
— pathological conditions arising from	191
— symptoms	189
— treatment	197
Peristalsis, effect of colonic contents on	17
— causes of	19
— experimental	17
— rate of	21
Peritoneum, abnormalities of, causing volvulus	78
— congenital abnormalities of	59
Peritonitis, adhesions following	93
— as a cause of acute dilatation	34
— general, following pericolitis	196, 199
Petroleum in chronic colitis	142
— chronic constipation	222
Physiology	13
— morbid	28
Polypi associated with other conditions	246
— cancerous	259
— malignant tendency	242
— multiple	237
— — symptoms	243
— — treatment	246
— predisposing to cancer	250, 253
Polypus as the starting-point of intussusception	117
Post-operative meteorism, causes of	35
Preparation of patient for operation	302
RE-ABSORPTION of water by the colon	13
Rectal bougies and tubes in diagnosis	55
Rectum, the normally empty state of	23
Resection and anastomosis of colon	302
— — multiple polypi	248
— — physiological results of	28
— of dilated colon	74
— entire colon, technique	316
— growths, restoring the bowel after	312
Reversal of colon, experiments in	23
Rupture of colon	276
SALINE infusion in operations	305
Sand, intestinal	25
Sarcoma	262
Segmentation	22
Sensory nerves	15

INDEX

	PAGE
Shiga's bacillus dysenteriæ in ulcerative colitis	156
Shock in operation, prevention of	305
Sigmoid flexure, anatomy of	9
—— cancer of	255, 270
—— on right side	60
Sigmoidoscopy, technique of	44
Simple stricture of the colon	233
— tumours	237
Spasmodic stricture of the colon	150
Splenic flexure, cancer of	269
Stercoliths in diverticula causing pericolitis	185
Stercolitis	228
Stercoral calculi	228
— ulcers	169
Stools, examination of	56
— in mucous colitis	130
Strauss's sigmoidoscope	44
Stricture of the colon, non-malignant	233
— following pericolitis	194
— polypi associated with	246
Symptoms, method of inquiry into	41
Syphilis	188
THROMBOSIS causing meteorism	32
— or embolism of blood-vessels	235
Toxins in obstructed bowel	26
Transverse colon, cancer of	255, 269
—— enteroptosis of	107
Traumatism	276
— a cause of pericolitis	188
Tropical dysentery and ulcerative colitis	154
Tubercle bacillus	40
Tuberculosis	201
— morbid anatomy	205
— hyperplastic	202
—— polypi associated with	246
— symptoms	209
— treatment	214
Tuberculous ulceration	172
Tumour formation from pericolitis	191, 199
—— — tuberculosis	204, 205
Tumours, simple	237

	PAGE
Tuttle's method of colotomy	283
Typhoid ulceration	177
ULCER, simple perforating	170
Ulceration causing pericolitis	188
— tuberculous	201
Ulcerative colitis	154
—— operative treatment of	173
—— perforation in	160
—— polypi associated with	246
Ulcers of colon, natural healing of	164
— distention or stercoral	169
Urine, examination of	57
VACCINE treatment of ulcerative colitis	172
Value cf the colon	14
Valve, ileocæcal	3
Vascular system	4
Veins, embolisms of colic	235
Venous thrombosis a cause of meteorism	32
Vesico-colic fistula following pericolitis	194
Vibration and massage in chronic constipation	224
Villous adenomata	237
Visceroptosis	107
Volvulus, acute, symptoms of	76
—— treatment of	87
— of cæcal angle	83
— chronic, symptoms of	77
—— treatment of	91
— compound	87
— etiology of	78
— pathology of	81
— prevention of recurrence of	89
Von Noorden's diet in chronic colitis	141
WATER, re-absorption by the colon	13
Witzel's operation for colotomy	283
Wounds of colon	276
X RAYS in diagnosis	51
— — — of chronic constipation	218
— — observation of peristalsis	19

RC860   L81

Lockhart-Mummery

Diseases of the colon.

RC 860   L81

CPSIA information can be obtained
at www.ICGtesting.com
Printed in the USA
LVHW040510290322
714677LV00003B/71